KT-569-835

3/02

T014247

04. NOV 02

05. JUN 03

08. DEC 03

05. JAN 04

16. FEB 04

23. APR 04

23. FEB

5 - APR 2012

OF01032

Books should be returned to the SDH Library on or before
the date stamped above unless a renewal has been arranged

Salisbury District Hospital Library

Telephone: Salisbury (01722) 336262 extn. 4432 / 33

Out of hours answer machine in operation

MANAGING AGGRESSION

Managing Aggression is a workbook designed for everyone who works in social care and anyone who has ever faced, or is likely to face, aggression at work. It provides a range of useful skills to help manage aggression, and shows staff placed in difficult and dangerous situations by their employees how to address the issue effectively by reducing the potential for violence. Individual chapters include:

Workplace culture * Causes of aggression * Assessing risk * Organisational responses to violence towards staff * Managing aggression * Bullying at work * Ethnic and gender issues * The consequences of aggression * Alternatives to aggression.

In examining the requirements of an employing agency to ensure its 'duty to care' for staff, *Managing Aggression* gives examples of good and bad practice and is packed with case studies and scenarios, charts and best-practice documents, learning objectives, activities to test knowledge and understanding, summaries of key learning points and key references.

Ray Braithwaite is a consultant and trainer in managing aggression and/or violence at work. He was a lead trainer and speaker in the national 'No Fear' campaign, aimed at reducing levels of violence towards social care staff, and has worked on local and central government bodies. He has published numerous articles on managing aggression in a range of professional journals and is the author of *Understanding Violence: Intervention and Prevention* (1992).

the social work skills series
published in association with *Community Care*

series editor: Terry Philpot

the social work skills series

- builds practice skills step by step

- places practice in its policy context

- relates practice to relevant research

- provides a secure base for professional development

This new, skills-based series has been developed by Routledge and *Community Care* working together in partnership to meet the changing needs of today's students and practitioners in the broad field of social care. Written by experienced practitioners and teachers with a commitment to passing on their knowledge to the next generation, each text in the series features: *learning objectives; case examples; activities to test knowledge and understanding; summaries of key learning points; key references; suggestions for further reading.*

Also available in the series:
Commissioning and Purchasing
Terry Bamford
Chair of the British Association of Social Workers and former Executive Director of Housing and Social Services in Kensington and Chelsea

Tackling Social Exclusion
John Pierson
Institute of Social Work and Applied Social Sciences, Staffordshire University

MANAGING AGGRESSION

Ray Braithwaite

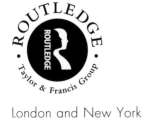

communitycare

London and New York

First published 2001
by Routledge
11 New Fetter Lane, London EC4P 4EE

Simultaneously published in the USA and Canada
by Routledge
29 West 35th Street, New York, NY 10001

Routledge is an imprint of the Taylor & Francis Group

© 2001 Ray Braithwaite

Designed and typeset in Sabon and Futura by Keystroke, Jacaranda Lodge, Wolverhampton
Printed and bound in Great Britain by TJ International Ltd, Padstow, Cornwall

All rights reserved. No part of this book may be reprinted or
reproduced or utilised in any form or by any electronic, mechanical,
or other means, now known or hereafter invented, including photocopying
and recording, or in any information storage or retrieval system, without
permission in writing from the publishers.

British Library Cataloguing in Publication Data
A catalogue record for this book is available from the British Library

Library of Congress Cataloging in Publication Data
Braithwaite, Ray, 1950–
Managing aggression / Ray Braithwaite.
p. cm. – (The social work skills series ; 1)
Includes bibliographical references and index.
1. Violence in the workplace. 2. Anger in the workplace. 3. Aggressiveness. I. Title. II. Series
HF5549.5.E43 B728 2001
650.1'3–dc21   2001019954

ISBN 0–415–24379–3 (hbk)
ISBN 0–415–24380–7 (pbk)

For Chris

CONTENTS

FIGURES

CASE STUDIES

SCENARIOS

INTERVIEW

ACKNOWLEDGEMENTS

With thanks to the London Borough of Croydon, Richmond-upon-Thames and East Sussex Social Services departments, the London Borough of Sutton Family Adolescent Support Team, and AWAKENS (Abused Women And Kids Everyone Needs Support), a project established by Domestic Violence Services (Keighley).

INTRODUCTION

Managing Aggression is a workbook designed for everyone who works in social care and for anyone who has ever faced, or is likely to face, aggression at work. The book is designed to give the reader a sense of empowerment by providing a range of useful skills which can help in managing aggression. More than this, however, the book also examines the requirements of the employing agency to ensure its 'duty to care' for staff, and gives the reader the means to address this issue in those agencies where staff are placed in difficult or dangerous situations.

In 1999 the magazine *Community Care* ran a campaign entitled 'No Fear' when it established that over half of those employed within social care had experienced aggression. This book is designed for all social care staff, with the ultimate aim being to help to substantially reduce violence to this staff force. After all, people are paid to do a job, they are not paid to be abused. This book examines examples of good and bad practice and provides numerous easy-to-use suggestions and solutions for reducing the level of aggression experienced by care workers.

The book is aimed at all social care staff whether they be field or residential social workers, day care staff, domiciliary workers or ancillary staff. It is equally aimed at the managers of these staff and sets out the responsibilities of the manager in ensuring that staff are safeguarded. Furthermore the book outlines the potential legal culpability involved for individuals and organisations failing to protect staff.

HOW TO USE THIS WORKBOOK

Each chapter is meant to stand alone and the reader is invited to start at the chapter most suited to him/her. If, however, you are using the book as the basis of a training programme, I would suggest the chapters be followed in sequence.

Throughout the book the reader will find case studies, questions and activities. These the reader is asked to consider and answer either individually or with other colleagues.

The workbook is valuable to the individual in helping them to both understand and manage aggression. It becomes a potentially more valuable tool when used within work-based teams where questions and issues regarding philosophy, attitudes and approach may be worked on jointly. The workbook may equally be used by trainers or others within a training session.

The National Task Force on Violence Against Social Care Staff defines violence as:

Incidents where persons are abused, threatened or assaulted in circumstances relating to their work, involving an explicit or implicit challenge to their safety, well-being or health.

(A Safer Place: Report of the Task Force and National Action Plan. Department of Health. Jan. 2001. www.doh.gov.uk/violencetaskforce)

Throughout this workbook the terms 'aggression' and 'violence' are used interchangeably.

CHAPTER 1

WORKPLACE CULTURE

This chapter considers different workplace cultures and their potential to affect the level of aggression experienced by staff. It will examine reasons why certain cultures are prevalent within social care and it will give the reader the opportunity to identify the culture that operates around them at work. The way that public opinion heightens the problems experienced in the work setting is also examined. Finally, measures that have brought about effective change in workplace cultures are identified to provide a suggested plan of action.

OBJECTIVES

By the end of this chapter you should:

- Have a clearer understanding of what the term 'violence' actually means within the workplace.

- Be aware of some of the negative cultures that are all too commonplace within social care.

- Have considered the element of 'zero tolerance' to aggression at work.

- Be able appropriately to challenge preconceived notions that aggression is 'a part of the job'.

- Identify ways of improving the public image of social care.

Figure 1.1 illustrates the points to be made and their interrelationship. Taking the workplace culture as the starting point, negative associations such as viewing aggression as inevitable become one of the barriers to effecting change. Bad practice may then be reinforced in a way that indirectly supports the continuation of violence; whereas strategies such as recording levels of abuse and clarity regarding sanctions break this circle.

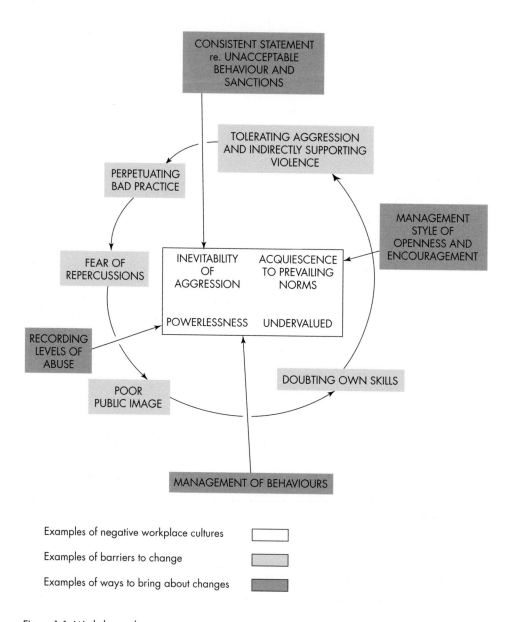

Figure 1.1 Workplace culture

THE CULTURE OF INEVITABILITY

At the start of any training course I usually pose the question: '*Have you experienced aggression within your work?*' At this stage many of the participants may not actually know what 'aggression' is. Some people think that aggression is purely physical, others that it involves either being purposefully damaged by another person or persons or having their lives put at risk. Some people think that an act is not really an aggressive act if it comes from someone who cannot understand what they are doing. Others think that 'they' (service users) have to do it as a means of expressing their frustration, and so, whatever the 'it' is, it is not categorised as aggression, even when this means that staff experience being scratched, pinched, spat at and so forth.

CONSIDER your workplace and the term 'aggression'.

Is there a certain level of aggression that staff are expected to tolerate? If so, why?

In order to attempt to focus course participants' thinking I prompt: '*I think you know when that line has been crossed. I think you know when you have experienced aggression.*' With this, usually between 80 and 100 per cent of participants answer 'Yes' to the question. Occasionally, however, one or two of the participants do not answer in the affirmative and for a brief moment my heart soars and, somewhat like the Heineken ad, I think 'How refreshing'. The moment does not last long, however, as the realisation of the answer that has been given sinks in. Instead of 'No' the typical alternative response is 'Not yet'. At this stage the group exchange knowing looks, a few people smile, perhaps remembering a time when they were new to the job before they had experienced aggression. One or two may even laugh and offer words of supposed comfort or encouragement, like '*Give it time*', to which the veterans in the group nod.

This culture of inevitability is endemic within some agencies and it is one that must be challenged and changed, otherwise it becomes a self-fulfilling prophecy. It is also probably a contributory ingredient to the fact that social care staff have the lead position in being the most abused profession as compared to any other comparable working group.[1]

ACTIVITY 1.1

In a group discuss:

Does your workplace have a culture of inevitability that aggression will occur?

No one is paid to be abused (verbally or otherwise), threatened, intimidated, shouted at, harassed, assaulted or murdered. Thankfully the murders are rare, yet the death of Jenny Morrison, a qualified, experienced and skilled worker, in November 1998 at the hands of a service user, plus the deaths of seven other social care staff since 1984, prove the risk is always with us. Aggression is not a part of the job and any workplace culture that implies that it is, is wrong.

ACTIVITY 1.2

In a group, brainstorm (or discuss):

1 In order to bring a halt to the 'culture of inevitability' what is required within my workplace is . . .

2 This can be achieved by . . .

Often new employees 'slot in' to the existing workplace culture and practices, accepting the 'norms' operating around them as good or at least standard practice for working with 'this client group'. Sometimes this may involve perpetuating approaches, attitudes and systems that are harmful to the service user. A clear example of this was identified in the MacIntire exposé shown on national television in November 1999. In this programme potentially harmful methods of physical intervention were identified as commonplace and regularly used within a residential establishment caring for people with learning difficulties. This was, it must be stressed, contrary to both the advice given by the Department of Health (DOH) concerning physical restraint and to good practice. The advice given by the DOH at that time emphasised that physical restraint was to be used as a last resort and must not become a regular feature of practice.[2]

Many of the staff who were filmed in the exposé would no doubt consider as wrong a regime that made use of the regular imposition of physical force as a means of achieving compliance by the service user, especially if such a regime were to be applied to them. Yet it was the staff in the unit who were the ones who perpetuated the regime, and new staff at best acquiesced and at worst became a part of the regime which considered frequent physical intervention to be 'acceptable practice' for this group of service users.

Why would staff go along with, or become part of such a regime?

This was an extreme case and, with the advent of the Public Interest Disclosure Act (1998) and the new regulations that came out in July 1999 safeguarding the whistle blower, the 'cover-up culture' should be a thing of the past. (Points regarding the Public Interest Disclosure Act are included at the end of this chapter.) However, at a less extreme level the experience of going along with the prevalent culture is not uncommon. Often we are clear in our private lives about what is and what is not acceptable behaviour. Yet this clarity is somehow changed, or lost, when it comes to the level of aggressive behaviour we will tolerate at work. At home, for instance, if someone were to tell us to '*fuck off*', generally the majority of us would regard that as unacceptable and we would probably do something about it. However, when we first walk into a new job, although we may initially be shocked at the levels of abusive language and behaviour prevalent, how many of us look around and, because other staff members are putting up with it, think to ourselves, '*That must be what I'm expected to put up with around here*'? In effect, we adapt to the implied negative workplace culture of acceptability and inevitability – rather than the positive one of 'This behaviour is unacceptable and it requires me and my colleagues to work with it in order to change it where possible.'

In order to bring about effective change to the culture of acquiescence all team members must have a clear starting point concerning the level of behaviour that they feel is acceptable and that which is unacceptable. Once behaviour is identified as unacceptable it becomes possible to manage, or attempt to manage, consistently.

STRATEGY: DEFINING 'VIOLENCE'

ACTIVITY 1.3

In a group of four to five people:

1 Make a brainstormed list of the Negative Words and/or Negative Behaviours you have experienced while doing your job. Please be specific when you describe the behaviour and words but do not, at this stage, give any information about the circumstances, or the age, gender or state of the person who behaved in this way.

2 Next, still in your group, think about the impact this behaviour or this word had upon you and write it down alongside. Think about the impact from three positions:

(a) How did you feel at the time?
(b) Did the situation have an impact upon your home life (irritability, inability to sleep, etc.)?
(c) Is there an ongoing impact of desensitisation?

Your list may now look something like this:

NEGATIVE WORDS/BEHAVIOURS	IMPACTS/EFFECTS
Told to 'fuck off'	Nothing. It happens all the time
Called a bastard. Bitch. Cow. Slag	Angry. Upset. Annoyed
Threatened with a knife	Sweating. Afraid. Shaken. Trembling
Spat at	Unclean. Disgust. Powerless. Angry
Brick thrown at me	Terrified. Valueless. Why me?
Finger in my face	Fear. Heart racing. Shock

continued

3   Now for the third and often hardest part of the exercise. Think of the individual circumstances. Think of the person whose behaviour you described. Think about what was going on in their life at the time they exhibited this behaviour. What was your part in this situation? What did you do, or say?

While you are thinking about the individual circumstances, AS A GROUP IDENTIFY (by placing a tick alongside) ANY of the above behaviours and/or words that the group considers to be ACCEPTABLE.

So if for example you think being 'spat at' is acceptable, perhaps because of the circumstances or condition of the person doing it, place a tick alongside that behaviour.

During this part of the exercise please discuss the difference between ACCEPTABLE and UNDERSTANDABLE behaviour.

4   Once this is completed, identify any of the behaviours that have been ticked. If there are any, identify the impact that the negative word or behaviour had upon the person concerned.

5   Now discuss:

(a) Is it acceptable for behaviour to damage another individual?
(b) If we do not address negative behaviour, what message are we giving to the person who is exhibiting that behaviour?
(c) What message are we giving to the other service users who may witness such behaviour?

We can see from the above that there is a difference between UNDERSTANDABLE and ACCEPTABLE behaviour and, whilst it remains fundamentally important to retain the quality of understanding, workers must not allow this quality of understanding to impair perception. Words or behaviours that damage another human being are simply UNACCEPTABLE and as such must be managed and not tolerated. If tolerated, the message provided to the service user is 'please continue'. Furthermore the message given to other service users who may witness the behaviour is equally negative.

It has long been recognised that individuals are unique and what may damage one may have no effect upon another. Individuals can be damaged by a word as well as a deed. This recognition was highlighted in 1992 when the Association of Directors of Social Services identified violence as: **'Behaviour which produces damaging or hurtful effects physically or emotionally on other people.'**

This definition does not limit violence to merely a physical injury. It states that the victim may be damaged emotionally, i.e. experience 'hurtful effects'. However, the hardest part of this definition for any of us to own up to, to identify and to report is the emotional impact that dealing with this behaviour may have generated within us.

ACTIVITY 1.4

Individually or within a group, brainstorm:

Why is being damaged emotionally the hardest part for any of us to report?

The reasons given for not reporting the emotional impacts often include:

> '. . . *viewed as a sign of weakness* . . . *my colleagues seem to put up with it so I think I should be able to* . . . *it's personal and I don't want my colleagues to know that I'm affected.* . . . *I don't want people to think I can't cope.* . . . *I want to preserve my self-image that I can manage* . . . *we're not supposed to have emotions, that's for the service user.* . . .'

In order to ensure accurate recording of the level of abuse and violence that staff are experiencing it is necessary to address the reasons for failing to report such events. Setting aside fears of being seen as failing to cope and the perception of staff that violence is inevitable because of the job, there is also the notion that staff are valued less than those they are employed to help.

THE 'A PART OF THE JOB' CULTURE

I am constantly amazed at the number of those staff who still sincerely believe that violence is a part of the job. Phrases like '*it goes with the turf*' and '*you've just got to cope with it*' are all too commonplace. Sometimes people believe that it is all right for someone who does not know better, by virtue of illness (e.g. dementia), state (e.g. learning difficulties) or tradition (it's the way they express themselves), to be aggressive. Not only is this belief patronising, but it is also potentially harmful to the service user and dangerous to the service provider. Such a belief precludes the opportunity to consider and then implement approaches to change the behaviour. The service user is labelled as 'unchangeable' and/or 'violent', or behaviour is identified as a part of the personality. Listen for phrases such as '*that's just him*' or '*she's like that*' or even '*you learn to expect that sort of thing from him/her*'. It is phrases like these which are often associated with excusing biting, scratching, pinching, punching, slapping, and so on.

When constantly under pressure from the full range of difficulties associated with caring for vulnerable people, it may seem easier to simply put up with the behaviour rather than to have to identify and then implement programmes to bring about changes to that behaviour. This becomes particularly pertinent in a system where financial constraints usually dictate service provision. Managers and staff soon learn that to push for additional resources, or perhaps more appropriate placement for the service user, can result in them being perceived as either causing trouble or lacking in appropriate professional skills.

In your workplace do you have any service users whose aggressive behaviour is tolerated rather than 'managed'?

Sometimes we excuse behaviour, identifying it as the by-product of an event or series of events beyond the control of the individual.

'It's not his/her fault, it's because ... he's unwell ... she's an old woman ... he's a person with learning difficulties ... he's suffering from dementia/Alzheimer's ... she's in care ... that's the way he is' ... and so on.

This approach creates a system that actually implicitly supports violence, as once again it fails to promote one that considers strategies for managing the behaviour. By precluding opportunities for 'treatment' of the behaviour at any level we let service users down and fail to ensure the health and safety of staff (see Chapter 3).

Another approach, which is often maintained, is to reward bad behaviour. Each of the following examples illustrates this not uncommon practice:

Example of behaviour	Action by staff/outcome
Drunken mentally ill client storms into the office without an appointment. Shouting abuse he threatens the receptionist and demands to be seen.	Queue-jumps and is seen by two social workers. Other clients have to wait even longer.
Female resident wants own room. Starts to bite staff, then scratch, then smear faeces on walls.	Given own room.
Service user makes complaints about home carer and threatens to 'take this further'.	Manager apologises and a new home carer is appointed.
Person fails to qualify for a service. Makes complaint to Director.	Staff directed to provide service.
Client with personality disorder says, 'I will kill myself if you don't . . .'	To date, staff have done whatever he asks.

ACTIVITY 1.5

In a group, identify:

At work, do staff reward bad behaviour? If so, how?

As in the example given above, list examples under the following headings:

Briefly describe the circumstances   **Actions taken by staff/outcome**

The difficulty in questioning existing regimes can be spotted immediately. Anyone employed within an organisation is unlikely to start questioning the fundamental make-up of the organisation for fear of losing their job or of being ostracised by their colleagues. Add to this the potential minefield of group dynamics, and the difficulties for the newcomer in challenging existing practices become even more pronounced. Imagine, for example, how resentful you would feel if you had been working within a system for some time, and then someone who may have only been employed for a few weeks started questioning the way you operated.

What systems are available to you and your colleagues to allow for the consideration of a change in work practice?

Unfortunately, all too often the person who does speak out can be the one who is ostracised by those operating the regime. Their ability may be questioned and often their working life can be made so intolerable that they feel forced to leave or they become totally demoralised.

CASE STUDY

Tracy had been in post for six months, working in a home for adolescent girls where violent incidents were a frequent occurrence. She recalls one night that was particularly bad. 'There had been a disturbance during the day when the police had interviewed a number of the older children about drugs on the estate where the home was sited. Two of the girls, Mandy (14 years) and Kim (15 years), had not liked being interviewed at all. Kim had stormed out of the session, throwing papers and knocking a table over. Mandy simply refused to be interviewed and started screaming at the male care officer who had gone to fetch her. Eventually, after the police had left, the place started to quieten down and we were able to get tea under way.

I was on that evening with Steve and we were expecting Doreen but unfortunately she phoned in sick. No one else had been called in, even though we knew the police would be calling. It was a fairly regular occurrence and though I'd been in touch with my manager about it, to forewarn her, no extra precautions had been suggested.

That night there were nine girls between the ages of 9 and 15 in the home. Usually they stay with us until they are about 16 but no more. Mandy and Kim were our oldest and they were inseparable. They were into everything on the estate, and frankly I thought they had something to do with the incident the police were investigating. After tea, Mandy and Kim went out, a couple of the other girls were watching the television in the lounge, and the rest were just sat around talking about what the police asked them. There was a lot of good-humoured giggling and things were settling down.

Then Mandy and Kim came back in a real state – angry and stomping around, disrupting everything and everyone. I went over to them to try to have a talk and calm them down a little. Mandy came at me and pushed me against the wall. I was so shocked. She might only be 14, but she's my size and much stronger than me. I just didn't know what to do. She held a needle close to my face and said something like, "This is what they were on about, you know." I thought she might, I don't know, maybe stick it in me. That was the worst part of it. It's the part I will always remember.

Fortunately, Steve had come out of the lounge to see what the noise was and he shouted something and Mandy let go. Then they both took off. I was really so shaken. Steve was very good but he had his hands full with looking after the other girls.

Nothing has changed in the home since this. Mandy and Kim are still terrorising everyone, staff included. No action has been taken regarding the incident. The general attitude of the staff is "there's nowhere else for Mandy and Kim to go to so their behaviour has to be tolerated".'

1 What would you do if you were Tracy?

2 How would you describe this workplace culture?

3 What changes are required and how could these be achieved?

In the above case study it is clear that attitudes must change to the way aggression is tolerated by default. Otherwise it may result in the macho stances often institutionalised by the same workers who, though hard pressed to survive themselves, unwittingly obstruct change by their sense of impotence often coupled with cynicism.

ACTIVITY 1.6

Break up into groups of up to five people and then spend up to one hour thinking through and making notes under the following headings:

1 AIMS AND OBJECTIVES OF THE WORKPLACE

2 WHAT IS YOUR WORKPLACE CULTURE?
   Words to describe   Examples to illustrate

3 WHAT SHOULD IT BE LIKE?
   Words to describe   Examples to illustrate

This exercise gives groups who work together the opportunity to identify positive changes to practice which can help both the worker and the service user. The following illustration may provide useful guidelines. It was completed by a group of staff who visit the homes of service users in order to teach the adult(s) how to play with their child(ren).

1 AIMS AND OBJECTIVES OF THE WORKPLACE
   To provide quality time to the child and parent
   To enable positive interaction between child and parent
   To give non-violent examples of disciplining/encouraging
   To help parent to develop social skills
   To reduce isolation

2 WHAT IS YOUR WORKPLACE CULTURE?

Words to describe	Examples to illustrate
Too busy watching your own back	Team meetings – afraid to say anything because picked off as troublemaker
Depressing, chaotic, tiring	Temporary accommodation – unsuitable

Uncaring about me – told to do it	Made to work with families that smoke – impact on my health. I should have a choice
Uncaring – contracts say 'flexitime'	Told you can't have it
Macho	Expected to go alone
Fearful	Told if you don't like it you can always leave

3   WHAT SHOULD IT BE LIKE?

Words to describe	*Examples to illustrate*
Supportive	Good teamwork. All talking openly about things
Good management	More training. Not defensive. Spend time talking with team members, not locked away in their offices
Should feel happy to go to work	One or two good-time events each year. To be told when you are doing a good job, not only told what you did wrong
Should feel secure	Told that the risks have been assessed and measures are in place. Told that it's OK to leave if I feel in danger

It was clearly very painful for the team to highlight the differences between the reality of their day-to-day experiences and the security/support to which they aspired, but by completing this exercise they were freed to use their current dissatisfactions to fuel their desire for change rather than have it continue to wear them down.

THE NO-VALUE CULTURE

The overall public impression of social care is not good and must be changed because it impacts upon the levels of aggression experienced by staff by:

- having a direct influence on staff morale
- devaluing the workers involved
- discouraging recruitment to the profession
- ultimately influencing resources

All too often the negative images of what goes wrong within social work/care are the only ones depicted. Bad practice highlighted in this way is then identified in the public mind as an example of standard practice throughout the service. This poor public image has an impact upon both morale and performance. I wonder for instance how many of us, when asked by a stranger, 'What do you do for a living?' would proudly reply 'I'm a social care worker'? Alternatively, how many of us fudge the answer with something like, 'I work with older people', or even 'I work in local government'?

At the performance level it appears that social care staff are constantly having to justify their existence and 'meet targets' or 'set appraisals' and obtain 'best value' with the drive to become more 'businesslike'. Whilst the aim to become more accountable is to be praised, it must be remembered that this is difficult to achieve in an arena of diminishing resources and increasing demand. The resource issue will not be resolved immediately. However, it is one that may be influenced positively if the public impression of social care could be improved.

IMPLEMENTING CHANGE
Influencing workplace culture at agency level

In order to bring about effective change to the workplace culture and obtain an accurate picture of the levels of abuse, aggression and violence staff are experiencing, many agencies are now attempting to ensure that *all* situations of aggression are officially recorded. Additionally, by giving clear guidelines identifying what staff are expected to report, the opportunity for local managers and individual workers to misinterpret policy is reduced. The London Borough of Croydon is clear in its policy statement, 'Coping with Violence Towards Staff':

> This strategy emphasises the Council's commitment to the protection and care of its staff in accordance with Health and Safety at Work Act 1974. It aims to minimise the risk of violence and give advice on the Council procedures to be followed. It also stresses the need to:
>
> - fully support staff who have suffered violence
> - view violence to staff as unacceptable and not 'part of the job'
> - treat all violent incidents seriously and act immediately

Besides using the definition of violence, '*behaviour which produces damaging or hurtful effects physically or emotionally on other people*', Croydon Council gives its staff specific examples of behaviours that are unacceptable and which are to be reported on its official 'Violence at Work Incident Form':

Types of violent behaviour

Harassment	Non-physical	Physical
Sexual	Verbal abuse (name-calling etc.)	Spiteful behaviour (e.g. spitting, pinching)
Racial	Verbal threats (e.g. 'I'll get you')	Physical attack without injury
Disability	Non-verbal threats (e.g. fist to face)	Physical attack with injury

The London Borough of Richmond-upon-Thames in its 'Safe Work with Clients – Code of Practice' statement is equally clear:

> Incidents of violence and aggression must be very carefully recorded (on the Incident Report Form).

Richmond also lists examples of behaviour to be recorded:

For the purposes of this code of practice, the following aspects of violent and/or aggressive behaviour are included:

Violence: the use of physical force against a person or object

Verbal abuse: the use of derogatory language or shouting aggressively

Threatening or intimidating behaviour: the use of actions or words in such a way as to coerce the victim or make them feel uncomfortable

Aggression: this can refer to either verbal or physical abuse

This code applies if staff are subjected to behaviour which, in their opinion, produces damaging or hurtful effects physically or emotionally on themselves or other people.

Even with these measures, under-reporting of violence remains at an unacceptably high level (see Chapter 4). One aim of the National Task Force on Violence Against Social Care Staff was to ensure a consistency in defining 'violence', as a means of increasing reporting, thereby providing a clearer identification of the levels experienced by care staff.[3] The definition provided by this group is given on page 2.

ACTIVITY 1.7

Discuss with your team:

Do you officially record on your INCIDENT FORM all incidents of abusive language, shouting, name-calling and threatening behaviour? If not, please identify the reasons why not.

Reasons often given for failing to officially record incidents include:

- I didn't know you could record just being shouted at
- Other staff don't record it so I thought it was something about me
- No one ever told me about the Incident Form
- If I filled in a form every time I was sworn at I'd be doing nothing else all day
- I thought you just recorded the physical things
- I don't want to get the service user into trouble

STRATEGY: THE CONCEPT OF ZERO TOLERANCE

Some agencies are going further. East Sussex County Council is currently investigating the possible use of a notice declaring zero tolerance of violence to staff strategically placed within some of its social services establishments. The notice clearly states:

East Sussex County Council Social Services Department WILL NOT TOLERATE ABUSIVE LANGUAGE OR VIOLENT BEHAVIOUR.

ACTIVITY 1.8

Individually consider, or within a group identify:

Reasons FOR and reasons AGAINST the use of a sign:

'THIS AGENCY WILL NOT TOLERATE ABUSIVE LANGUAGE
OR BEHAVIOUR'.

Generally the arguments used concerning the use of such a sign include:

For	Against
A clear message, allowing people to know where they stand	Makes people think about being violent
	Provocative
Supportive of staff	Creates fear
Reassuring to less powerful clients	Expectation that it will happen
Staff can point to it and alleviate the need for discussion	Implies sanctions
Sets clear boundaries	Gets ignored
Supportive of other non-violent/non-abusive service users	People don't read notices
	It won't work

Such zero tolerance signs have been valuable in a variety of other venues and can presently be seen in some public houses in the form, 'IF YOU ARE ABUSIVE OR OFFENSIVE TOWARDS A MEMBER OF STAFF OR ANOTHER MEMBER OF THE PUBLIC THE POLICE WILL BE CALLED AND YOU WILL BE BANNED', or more simply, 'NO DRUGS. NO VIOLENCE'. They can also be found in football stadiums, hospitals and in many public transport arenas.

STRATEGY: SANCTIONS

The sign will not work in its own right and it must be backed up with the potential for a sanction to be imposed if it is not adhered to. One of the principal values of such a sign is that it forces the agency using it to actually clarify what sanctions it can or will take, should the need arise. This becomes particularly relevant, especially as a major issue in relation to violence towards social care staff is the apparent lack of any action taken against the perpetrator of the aggressive act. Sanctions do not have to be major, but they must be available.

ACTIVITY 1.9

Individually or in a group:

Identify what sanctions are available in your work to help manage aggressive behaviours?

Sanctions can range from the appropriate use of time – 'You have just been shouting at me, I will not see you for thirty minutes' – to the ultimate sanction of withdrawing a service, where appropriate. The London Borough of Croydon, for example, in its corporate policy states:

> The council is committed to using legal action to prevent violence to its staff and deter the violent customer. The legal department will, on behalf of the council, institute criminal proceedings following the abuse of or an assault upon an employee (subject to evidence).

Such actions become possible under Section 222 of the Local Government Act, 1972, where a local authority considers it appropriate 'for the promotion or protection of the interests of inhabitants of their area'. Similarly, there is scope for local authorities to issue civil proceedings in their own right in order to protect the interests of a significant number of staff. Other agencies take the approach of sending a solicitor's warning letter to violent or potentially violent service users, while others may exclude the user from the service (see also Chapter 9).

The use of a formal sign is equally valid in providing a clear and unequivocal message on behalf of the organisation that violence and aggression are not acceptable and are not to be considered 'a part of the job'.

INFLUENCING WORKPLACE CULTURE – INDIVIDUAL LEVEL

Many social care staff believe that the workplace culture is established by the Director and the senior management of the department or agency. Furthermore they believe that the policies of the agency give a clear indication of the way staff are valued. However, the individual workplace culture is often influenced at a more local level.

Consider the impact upon a team of the following (not untypical) comments made by administrative and support staff at training sessions:

> They seem to think they are better than us – most of the social workers use the 'f' word in my office, I don't like it but what can I do? – at the interview I was told to expect aggression from one of the senior managers – it happens all the time. They [social workers] get frustrated and I get shouted at.

It is important that all staff are included within a caring regime and that we should respect equally those with different roles. Openness and positive communication styles are imperative to the workplace culture, and teams must pay due respect to the way communication takes place throughout.[4]

One factor often given as a reason for not disclosing information to our work colleagues is that of CONFIDENTIALITY. However, confidentiality does not preclude staff safety which is paramount in law.

Another influential factor establishing the workplace culture is the local manager. Individual managers often place individual interpretation upon the levels of violence they expect their staff to tolerate. The reasons for this include:

- not wanting too many reports completed, as the impression given is that the manager is failing to do their job
- over-focusing upon meeting the needs of the clients/service at all costs
- the need to meet targets to prove viability, etc.
- the '"macho" staff should be able to put up with this sort of thing', approach
- the unawareness of the overall policy

This reinforces the need for agencies to have clear guidelines accessible to all workers for recording incidents of violence.

INFLUENCING PUBLIC OPINION

Although the issue of under-resourcing is not likely to be influenced directly, it could be influenced positively if the public impression of social care were to be improved. Other positive outcomes of a good public image may include the recruitment and retention of more staff to the profession and the retention of existing staff, as well as improvements to the morale and ultimately the performance of those staff presently within social care. In order to be achieved, however, this change in perception must be attempted both at an organisational and at an individual level. Organisationally agencies can:

- ensure that good communication between local press and media is established in order that events promoting the image of social care can be highlighted
- publish their own 'good news' in newsletters, periodicals, etc.
- promote the positive aspects of social care at a national level
- prove they value staff by providing appropriate facilities
- provide regular developmental as well as task-focused supervision for staff
- ensure enough staff are available to do the job expected

Individually much can be done to improve the image of the social care resource that is provided locally. Teams can:

- identify and promote good practice
- identify imaginative ways of involving the local community
- organise developmental meetings to augment the 'task-focused' ones
- positively praise individuals for achievements
- spend time considering staff morale and ways of improving it where necessary

ACTIVITY 1.10

As a team, brainstorm the following:

What can be done in your workplace to help improve your image?

CONCLUSION

Workplace culture fundamentally influences levels of aggression experienced by staff. Get the culture right and levels of aggression experienced and the often disabling high levels of stress generated from the aggression will diminish. Get it wrong and they will remain high.[5]

The workplace culture that reduces the level of aggression:

- offers a clear commitment to staff that violence at work is unacceptable
- has a policy and procedure on violence at work which is known by all staff
- has a simple user-friendly incident reporting form
- takes a proactive stance to ensure that incidents do not occur
- provides appropriate sanctions to perpetrators of violence
- has a usable definition
- actively monitors all acts of aggression to identify trends, dangerous environments or dangerous people
- takes appropriate action to stop recurrence
- treats all acts of aggression towards staff seriously
- does not minimise aggressive acts
- provides legal advice for staff subjected to violence, informing them of their rights
- provides personal insurance for staff and compensation for those subjected to violence
- ensures that comprehensive support is available via counselling and appropriate debriefing
- provides training for staff on methods of managing aggression
- proactively promotes a positive public image
- believes that staff are the most important commodity the agency has and manages them as such

KEY POINTS

This chapter should have challenged some previously held perceptions that violence is 'a part of the job'. It should have given you some ways to challenge that and other preconceived ideas possibly held by your colleagues.

REMEMBER:

- ☐   You are not paid to be abused. You are paid to do a job.
- ☐   Violence associated with work is unacceptable.

- ☐   It should not be considered 'a part of the job' or put down to 'their way'.
- ☐   Violence needs to be managed not tolerated.
- ☐   The culture of the workplace is a fundamental factor to take into account when attempting to address the issue of violence at work.
- ☐   REPORT all incidents of violence and abuse no matter how trivial they may seem.

Further information about the Public Interest Disclosure Act 1998 can be obtained from the Department of Trade and Industry: 1 Victoria Street, London SW1H 0ET (website: www.dti.gov.uk).

---

1   New law designed to protect workers who blow the whistle on malpractice(s).

2   Aimed at promoting greater openness between bosses and their workers.

3   Prior to the legislation, research suggested that about 80 per cent of whistle blowers lost their jobs.

4   Now any dismissal on the grounds of 'whistle blowing' is automatically considered unfair; irrespective of length of service, workers become 'protected'.

5   Does not provide workers with a charter to spread gossip.

6   Only covers those disclosures that the worker reasonably believes show malpractice related to criminal offences; failure to comply with legal obligations; miscarriages of justice; danger to health or safety or damage to the environment, or any 'cover-ups' related to these.

7   Disclosure is to be made in good faith.

8   Act encourages employers and workers to deal with matters internally, except in more extreme circumstances, by establishment of an 'authorised person' to whom disclosure may be made.

9   There is scope for some disclosures to be made to someone other than the employer or authorised person. For instance some workers may be protected if they make disclosure to Government ministers or a person prescribed by the Secretary of State.

10   Media involvement may preclude 'protection' for staff members if not disclosed to authorised person or employer beforehand – unless by doing so they would be victimised.

11   Any employee who makes a disclosure for personal gain would not be protected.

12   Intended to end 'cover-up culture'.

13   Compensation for whistle blowers who are unfairly dismissed will not be subject to a monetary limit.

Figure 1.2 Points regarding Public Interest Disclosure Act 1998

REFERENCES

1   National Institute for Social Work (NISW) Briefing Number 26 (Oct. 1999) which gives an overview of the literature on violence and abuse of staff, the findings from NISW Social Services Workforce Studies on violence, and local authority and other organisational policies and guidelines. May be obtained from: National Institute for Social Work, 5 Tavistock Place, London WC1H 9SN. (website: www.nisw.org.uk or info@nisw.org.uk).

2   *Guidance on Permissible Forms of Control in Children's Residential Care* (1993). Issued by the Department of Health. HMSO. Information available at Department of Health (website: www.doh.gov.uk).

3   *A Safer Place: Combating Violence Against Social Care Staff*. Report of the Task Force and National Action Plan. Department of Health. Jan. 2001 (www.doh.gov.uk/violencetaskforce).

4   Whittaker, D., Archer, L. and Hicks, L. (1998) *Working in Children's Homes: Challenges and Complexities*. Wiley; and Balloch, S., McLean, J. and Fisher, M. (eds) (1999) *Social Services: Working Under Pressure*. Policy Press.

5   See 3 above.

KEY READING

Fletcher, K. 'Managing the media.' *Community Care*. 24 Feb.–1 March 2000.

Heller, R. (1998) *Managing Teams*. Dorling Kindersley.

Holihead, M. 'Whistleblowing.' *Community Care*. 20–26 Jan. 2000.

Humphries, J. (1998) *Managing Successful Teams: How to Achieve Your Objectives by Working Effectively with Others*. How to Books.

No Fear Campaign: weekly contributed articles. *Community Care*. 22 July–Dec. 1999.

Taylor, G. (1999) *Managing Conflict*. Directory of Social Change, 24 Stevenson Way, London NW1 2DP.

CHAPTER 2

CAUSES OF AGGRESSION

Aggression for many of us is either the outward expression of an internal emotion or an action created by circumstance. For a small minority, however, there is no root cause generating the behaviour. A small minority of the people you will come into contact with will use aggression in a cold, calculating manner to achieve their ends. For this minority, aggression will either be a part of their personality or it will be an element used as a manipulative tool. For the majority, however, aggression is a behaviour generated by a cause. As workers we can more effectively manage aggressive behaviour, therefore, by determining those causes. Once identified we may then concentrate on attempting to eliminate some of these causes from our work. It becomes a simple equation: reduce the causes that are giving rise to the behaviour and we will reduce the number of aggressive acts facing us.

OBJECTIVES

This chapter will:

- Identify a range of theoretical frameworks which place aggression in particular contexts.

- Consider some of the elements that may create aggressive behaviour.

- Identify those elements over which we have some control.

- Provide ideas for reducing levels of aggression currently facing you in your work.

By the end of the chapter you will be aware of some of those elements in work style, work environments, working practice(s), attitudes and approaches which increase the potential for aggression. Furthermore you will be able to identify changes required in these areas in order to reduce the potential for aggressive acts.

There are many theories about the causes of aggression and some of the following brief descriptions may help to order our thinking. This is by no means a comprehensive list. I have only provided the briefest of theoretical interpretation as a means of starting this chapter, because I want the chapter to be based in practice and you to consider practical ideas that can help reduce the potential for aggression taking place within your work. At the end of the chapter is a reading list for reference.

The natural or innate theory considers aggression to be a natural part of every human, as it is a part of every animal on earth. This theory suggests that as humans we must be the most aggressive of all the animal kingdom because we have effectively destroyed our competitors to achieve the dominant species position. Furthermore, we are now continuing in this need to dominate by destroying ourselves in warfare. All animals fight. However, human beings are the only species on earth who will fight over an idea, a belief or a religion. The positive aspect of this theory is that aggression is used by humans to survive difficult situations – we 'fight off' an illness, for example. It is a part of the competitive urge. It is a force that enables us to overcome difficult challenges in life.

The frustration theory argues that people become aggressive when their needs are not met, and aggression is a way of relieving the frustration generated within the body. Frustration is believed to be relieved, or, at least, temporarily dissipated, once the aggressive act is over.

The behavioural theory indicates that aggression is a learned process and will flourish within circumstances that reward the behaviour. This theory puts forward the view that behaviour is controlled by past experience and the consequences derived from those experiences. If the aggressor achieves his/her aims from the use of verbal or physical force, or its threat, the behaviour is reinforced, and from the perception of the aggressor there is no incentive to change.

Ecological theories argue that behaviour is affected by the conditions in which we live, and some experiments have identified that people will fight each other if food, air or space is scarce. This theory indicates that the environment can influence mood. Overcrowding, poor lighting, shabby furniture, enclosed spaces, noise and the enforced use of shared inadequate facilities are all arguments used by ecologists as causes of aggressive behaviour.

Sociological theories identify the causes of aggression as cultures, roles and stereotypes created by and within society. The still populist idea that men must be 'macho' and women 'feminine' places individuals under a lot of pressure to conform to this. The racist assumption that black people are somehow less intelligent than white can lead to a society that, by devaluing one set of human beings, creates strife as it provokes demands for justice from those so devalued. The potential for conflict is increased in a society that bases the distribution of resources upon stereotypical norms, thereby distributing those resources unequally.

Psychodynamic theories indicate that we are influenced by our past and the ways others related to us. If as children we were constantly told we were bad, naughty or not as good as our sibling(s), this can grow within the child to overwhelming proportions. As children we cannot express this feeling because most children do not have the skills to do so appropriately. When it is expressed it is often perceived as rebelling, thereby confirming the statements of our 'badness'. Anger is often therefore bottled up, sometimes for years, until it explodes in violent temper outbursts. Alternatively, as adults it is redirected towards someone who may remind us of a childhood protagonist; or even towards a group of individuals who may have some significance – classically authority figures.

The interactive theory suggests that aggressive behaviour is a process influenced by others. The theory proposes that if we are hostile to another person this can create aggression within them, which can lead to aggressive acts being perpetrated, thereby validating our initial hostility. It becomes a vicious circle. In this way, for instance, hostile acts by a service user may lead to a hostile response by the care worker. The aggressive client can therefore create a hostile environment which will in turn make them more hostile.

Chemically induced theories propose the concept that chemicals change behaviour and that some chemicals can induce aggression. These chemicals may be introduced externally in such forms as alcohol and drugs, or internally during physical illness, or at times of hormonal imbalance. The idea that some foodstuffs contain toxins which can cause aggression is popular and indeed is one which has given rise to some drinks and foods being removed from sale.

Alternatively the chemical change can be induced within individuals by circumstance. At times of trauma and stress the body experiences a surge of chemicals such as adrenaline, noradrenaline, cortisone and endomorphs from the adrenal gland. This is often referred to as the 'adrenaline buzz', and can be identified within some workers who like to 'get things going' in order to stimulate the adrenaline rush within themselves.

Added to the above, certain behaviours combine aspects of the different theories – take, for example, the **'mindless violence'** myth and the **'protective urge'**. The myth of 'mindless violence' was popularised especially during the 1980s and 1990s. Found as banner headlines in certain newspapers it was an attempt to give reason to the violent clashes between opposing sets of so-called football supporters. The myth suggests the idea of spontaneity, whereas in reality this form of aggression is usually planned and orchestrated. It is frequently xenophobic or homophobic in its base and performed by individuals operating within a group. It is therefore influenced by group processes with such elements as peer pressure, competition, the need to save face, and the desire to be identified as one of the group. Individually the perpetrator will often derive a reward for the behaviour, either in terms of payment by the organiser for the job done, or from the status gained within their peer group – or simply from the 'adrenaline rush' achieved.

The 'protective urge' highlights the need within many of us to defend those less able. This is very common within relationships where one person feels responsibility for another, and operates when the second person is at risk. Although prevalent within relationships it can also exist where injustice is being perpetrated towards a group or an individual perceived as less able to defend or speak up for themselves. It can include the desire or need to campaign on diverse issues such as 'rights of way' or global warming on behalf of those less able, articulate, aware or willing. It can also include the need/desire to protect animals and objects, especially those objects considered valuable in the perception of the protector.

ACTIVITY 2.1

Individually or in a group:

1 Consider the above theories and identify those that may be taking place within your workplace.

2 Give examples.

IDENTIFYING THE CAUSES

Most forms of aggression require a cause before they can occur. Think about it from your own perception. Is it easy for you to actually damage another person without cause? Provided with a cause we can more readily attack.

For the sake of example, imagine you are walking along a street and that you have a child with you who is about eight years old. Let us say that this is your child, or a relative's child, someone you feel responsible for. A man you do not know walks across the road, grabs the child and starts to shake the child in front of you. What would you do?

The majority of us would react instinctively by striking out, especially if we act in a protective capacity. We, in effect, are provided with a cause which creates our behaviour. This is of course an oversimplification. However, assuming that such an action as this can create aggressive behaviour within others, it becomes valuable to identify other, perhaps equally simplistic, 'causes' that may be taking place around us in our work styles, environments, systems, practices and/or attitudes and approaches. Once identified we can then begin to manage, and perhaps eradicate, some of these causes, and in this way we can make the theories on aggression work for us.

ACTIVITY 2.2

In a group:

1 Draw a line down the middle of a sheet of paper. Then on one side brainstorm:

What causes you to feel or become aggressive? (List at least ten elements/factors.)

2 Next, in the other column:

Give examples relating each of your listed points to your work.

Your list may look something like this:

What causes me to feel or become aggressive?	Examples related to work
1 Injustice	Caving into aggression

2	Being let down	Not backed up by management
3	Feeling someone is deliberately trying to put me down	Manipulative service users or people who treat me like a servant
4	Having something taken from me	My dignity (see above)
5	Invasion of territory	No safe space
6	Not being given relevant information	Not told if client has a history of violence
7	People being offensive towards me	Being sworn at every day
8	Attitude	Rudeness – little thanks – lots of criticism
9	Being kept waiting	Never knowing when transport will arrive
10	Inefficiency	Staff not doing what they say they will do

Let us consider each of these in turn and in particular how they may be applicable to our service users and the situations facing them.

1 Injustice. *Caving into aggression*

Within social care many acts of injustice take place on a regular basis, yet some of those injustices may be within our power to manage better.

> In your reception area a person is waiting to see you to talk to you about a relative. S(h)e has been quiet, undemanding and has been waiting for over fifteen minutes. You have sent a message to this person via the receptionist saying that you will not be very much longer, but that was about ten minutes ago and you have been caught up answering the telephone ever since. Now a really irate service user storms in demanding to see you. This person has a history of being aggressive if they do not get their own way. The receptionist is afraid of this person and has asked you to do something as quickly as possible to avoid the situation 'getting worse'.

What would you do?

Many of us would, unfortunately, see the irate, demanding service user first, so giving:

(a)   the service user the reinforcement that bad behaviour gains rewards

(b)   the person waiting a demonstrative model that they may consider using next time

ACTIVITY 2.3

Individually identify or in a group discuss:

In the above scenario what alternative methods are available to the care worker to better manage the behaviour?

There are a variety of approaches that could better manage the situation. These include:

1   clear boundaries about unacceptable forms of behaviour together with information concerning this which is given to service users
2   appropriate sanctioning of such behaviour (both-these ideas are covered more fully in Chapter 4)

Within social care other forms of injustice abound.

*   two workers are allocated to the person with the aggressive history while other service users have their service cut or reduced
*   some service users have their rights to liberty infringed as the door of the establishment is locked to prevent wandering by other less able-minded residents
*   people are left in bed or in their rooms longer than appropriate, waiting for the overworked staff member to get them up or out
*   day-care bus/transport arrives so late that it makes day care irrelevant
*   staffing ratios of one staff member to ten or more residents or day-care attendees provide little opportunity to allow for individual consideration
*   meal, bed and other important times are at the convenience of the worker and not within the power of the individual to influence
*   user choice is limited by availability – the ultimate choice usually being take it or leave it
*   inappropriate placement of a service user as a means of saving money means that their disruptive behaviour disadvantages other residents
*   user empowerment is considered poor practice by managers, and workers are criticised for 'provoking' action or blamed when action has no effect.
*   misinformation is provided by an agency to promote image at the expense of honesty

ACTIVITY 2.4

Identify any areas of INJUSTICE occurring within your workplace.

What can be done to address these?

2 Being let down. *Not backed up by management*

Sometimes a service user will use aggressive or offensive behaviour as a means of attempting to obtain a service or increase their priority for the service. At these times the care worker may well refuse to deal with the person concerned. It now becomes important to ensure that the aggressor does not receive special treatment or consideration from a more senior member of staff. The significance of this is increased when the service user proceeds to make a complaint about their 'treatment', while demanding to be dealt with by 'someone in authority'. All too often, unfortunately, a senior member of staff will cave in to the demands of the service user in order to keep the peace. This approach only reinforces the aggressor's behaviour and helps to demoralise staff. Furthermore, the aggressor is then able to return to her/his home environment spreading the news about how using aggressive tactics obtains a service or resource from that agency.

Now, consider this concept of 'being let down' from the perception of the service user. How many times do we let service users down? It may be a broken promise – *'I'll get back to you later in the day'* – being too preoccupied to listen – *'that's nice, dear'* – or simply being too busy to have the time to be aware of and make significant the special events in their life?

ACTIVITY 2.5

In a group:

1 List those occasions when you, your agency or the system have let the service user down.

2 Discuss:

What did you learn from that event?

---

3 Feeling someone is deliberately trying to put me down. *Manipulative service users or people who treat me like a servant*

Attempting to influence an outcome within a situation may well be acceptable. However, manipulation whereby we attempt to achieve our goals by devious or even harmful means is not. There are a variety of ways of being destructively manipulative: we can withhold information; concentrate on the negative aspects of the person and highlight these on every occasion; lie or misrepresent; misuse power; intimidate; use emotion inappropriately; fail to communicate appropriately; fail to treat the individual as an individual; patronise; purposefully antagonise; laugh at the person and give them no power over their situation. For our part we can learn to spot these behaviours and manage them (see Chapter 5). However, for our service user perhaps we need to identify and then challenge the behaviour on their behalf or, wherever possible, provide them with the skills to do so themselves.

ACTIVITY 2.6

In a group, draw a line down the middle of a sheet of paper. In the first column brainstorm:

How do staff wind service users up?

Next, in the second column, identify:

What can be done in you workplace to address each of the items on your list?

---

4 Having something taken from me. *My dignity*

Imagine the indignity at the loss of independence which must accompany many people who at the end of a productive life suddenly find themselves no longer able to cope. Add to this the need to suddenly adapt to group living and even to sharing a bedroom with a stranger who may well be incontinent. This may be further enhanced by staff assuming an automatic right to call the new resident by their first name – '*It's one of the rules here, Maisie. We think it's really friendly*' – even though the person concerned may consider the use of a title (Mr, Miss, etc.) as part of their identity and worth.

Sometimes we demonstrate how little we value our service users in what we provide for them.

SCENARIO

I called to see the social worker to talk about my mother. She'd been visited by them the day before and was really in a bit of a state. They said she couldn't cope and shouldn't be left alone. So I wanted to have a word with them about it and about what could be done. When I got there I was asked to wait. The person behind the desk was a bit shirty, expected me to know that I couldn't just turn up and expect to be seen. All I knew was they'd left a card with mom and it said to get in touch, so I did. Anyway I was told they'd get a duty officer to see me, so that was something.

To be honest the waiting room was not a pleasant place to wait in. There were two old armchairs that were ripped and stained with I don't know what and two kids were sprawled in them anyway. The orange plastic seats, those stacker ones, were as bad and when I sat down I sat on something sticky. The place smelt of stale and dirt and someone had sprayed air freshener but it didn't mask it. A young woman who looked like a tramp had a very dirty baby on her knee in the corner. The baby was crying and needed changing and the kids kept on making up jokes about it and about the young woman. Someone, maybe one of the social workers, had thought to bring in some old toys, dolls and things, for the kids I suppose, and these were all over the place. They might have been all right in their time but not any more. They just needed slinging. It looked really weird with these broken dolls left around. I couldn't stay and said to the woman behind the counter that I'd be outside having a smoke.

ACTIVITY 2.7

Individually or in a group, consider:

1 What could have been done better in the above scenario?

2 The potential effect upon you if you were forced to wait for a service in such an environment.

3 Do any such arenas exist within your workplace?

4 What is required to change this?

Ecologists would argue that aggressive behaviour would be more prevalent within environments that:

- are enclosed
- provide limited exits – one way in/one way out
- are monotone in colour
- are coloured a tone that is either non-uplifting – e.g. grey, brown, etc. – or is stark and vivid, such as white, yellow, orange, etc.
- have poor or no exterior light
- have stark interior lighting (strip) or dim lighting
- are graffitied or generally uncared for
- are dirty, noisy, smelly

5 Invasion of territory. *No safe space*

The majority of us need defendable space. This may be a room that can be locked, allowing a place for staff to retreat to if necessary, or an exclusive area away from the service user, providing a sanctuary helping to increase the feeling of security. However, defendable space is also an invisible area around ourselves which provides a sense of security. How big that space is depends upon situations and cultural norms. It is further influenced by gender, ethnic and religious circumstances, and it is therefore difficult to be prescriptive. However, a general rule concerning safety and space is:

> THE AVERAGE SPACE REQUIRED BETWEEN YOU AND AN AGGRESSOR SHOULD BE APPROXIMATELY TWO ARMS' LENGTH.

This amount of space is generally considered enough to allow you and the aggressor to feel less on edge, and it will give you enough opportunity to avoid a fist should one be used. It is a rule to be considered when standing, in a non-confrontational manner; if sitting, this may be relaxed to about one-and-a-half arms' length at head level, once again taking into account non-confrontational positioning. (For more information, see Chapter 5: Part A.)

Another general rule concerning defendable space is:

DO NOT TOUCH THE AGGRESSIVE PERSON FIRST

Even though your need may be to comfort, contain or control, that is your need. The need of the aggressor, who is acting on instinct, is not to be touched. If you touch the aggressor at this time you will generally release a trigger mechanism within that person which will allow him/her to touch you back about fifty times easier and fifty times harder than you touched them.

What form of invasion would cause you to react aggressively?

Be aware that although some agencies have areas designated solely for staff, and use coded locks and other devices to restrict entry, often the door is left open or toilet facilities are on the wrong side, so the idea of safety can be an illusion.

6 Not being given relevant information. *Not told if client has a history of violence*

Information is power, yet frequently it is withheld. The reasons for this vary.

* Sometimes it is mistrust – '*If I told them the truth they probably wouldn't admit him*'
* Sometimes it is pressure of work – '*I can't get all the paperwork done*'
* sometimes it is patronising – '*I really thought it was better for them if they weren't told*'
* Sometimes it is fear – '*I live in the area where I work and if I passed on what I knew he'd know where it came from*'

For whatever reason, withholding information is an abuse of power.

Are there any occasions when it is acceptable to withhold information?

In order for a comprehensive risk assessment to be completed under the health and safety legislation (see Chapter 3) it is vital that all relevant information about the service user concerned is made available to the individual staff member who is to have dealings with them. Under the legislation any person who fails to provide relevant information is effectively culpable and may become subject to the penalties contained within the legislation.

Frequently the argument of *confidentiality* is given as a reason for withholding information. This argument cannot justifiably be used where staff safety is concerned as:

- staff safety is paramount
- confidentiality is to the agency and not the individual worker

The argument of *confidentiality* is also dangerous as it may lead to a collusive and divisive approach. The difficulty may exist, however, in situations where information is contained in data form and where the principles of the Data Protection Act[1] must be adhered to (see Figure 2.1). An added difficulty may arise where information is required by other agencies involved. However, the same rule applies – individual worker safety is paramount, and the fact that the information is contained on computer does not preclude the passing on of relevant information pertinent to safety and risk.

Anyone processing personal data must comply with the following rules. The data must be:

- fairly and lawfully processed
- processed for limited purposes
- adequate, relevant and not excessive
- accurate
- not kept longer than necessary
- processed in accordance with the data subject's rights
- secure
- not transferred to countries without adequate protection

Personal data may cover both facts and opinions. It also includes information regarding the intentions of the use of the data, although in some limited circumstances exemptions will apply.

Figure 2.1 Principles of data protection

Ways and means must be identified to enable the passing on of appropriate information, and some agencies are currently examining how this may be achieved. One example of good practice, in identifying and passing on information, was a protocol published in October 1999 for use within Hampshire, Portsmouth, Southampton and the Isle of Wight.[2] This outlined a system for sharing information about potentially dangerous offenders.

Fear is often a cause generating aggression, and providing information is one way of helping to reduce that fear. Without information prejudice is rife. Prejudice with power leads to oppression, and one way to oppress is to withhold information. It becomes a vicious circle.

ACTIVITY 2.8

In a group identify:

What information do you withhold from your service users?

Discuss your reasons.

It is important how the information is both recorded and provided, so that the worker is able to make use of it. Generalised statements often generate increased powerlessness and therefore more fear. For example, statements like '*He can be violent*' or '*She has violent outbursts*' do little other than promote fear.

In order for the information to be valuable and usable it must:

- be a clear description of behaviour – what it was and at whom it was directed
- indicate the possible causes or triggers for the behaviour – immediate factors prior to the event, including the time of day etc.
- identify what was done to manage the behaviour and whether the approach was successful or not
- attempt to identify any repetitive recurrence of the behaviour
- say what happened next – such as was the behaviour sanctioned? Was the relationship with the service user renegotiated?

7 People being offensive towards me. *Being sworn at every day*

We often want to give as good as we get, or at least it is not unnatural to have that feeling. Social care workers face more abusive language, offensive and aggressive behaviour than any other comparable professional group.[3] It must equally be the case, therefore, that social care staff have the opportunity and desire to retaliate, more than any other professionals. It is not possible, desirable or professional to be aggressive. However, if, as the innate theory indicates, the natural instinct is to retaliate, being 'professional' and 'learning to cope' must often create a lot of internal stress, confusion and anger for the care worker. In this atmosphere, therefore, it becomes imperative that care workers are given appropriate time to debrief. Unfortunately, at times of financial constraint, debriefing sessions are cut, staff development time is decimated and supervision sessions become solely task-focused. The individual worker is often left to find their own resources for debriefing, or has to do without.

ACTIVITY 2.9

Think through, or in a group discuss:

What form of debriefing is required in an environment where staff are regularly verbally abused?

The culture of an establishment is crucial, and it will either maintain or attempt to reduce the level of violence experienced by staff. In those situations where staff are experiencing being regularly verbally abused, the organisation must be prepared to act to bring a halt to the abuse. If it fails to do so, the organisation itself may be responsible for creating an environment where staff and service users become locked into a culture of violence.

8 Attitude. *Rudeness – little thanks – lots of criticism*

There are a variety of ways of being rude. We may:

- ignore the person and talk to our colleague while attending to them
- talk about them in their presence to another
- be abrupt, offhand or curt, or alternatively remain silent yet grumpy
- deny their emotions or their situation
- turn away
- use a tone of voice that implies disbelief or incredulity
- be superior or arrogant
- patronise
- exclude

One way of doing this is to use a particular form of code known by an exclusive group – jargon. Within social care jargon is rife, ranging from phrases such as '*Domiciliary assessment*', '*care package*', '*case conference*', etc., to the ever popular '*I hear what you are saying*', '*I can see where you are coming from*', or even '*I can feel your pain*', and so on. It includes the use of letters and numbers – e.g. *SSI*, *DGM* and *SS21* – as well as important-sounding words – e.g. '*numeracy level*' or '*symbiotic relationship*'. There is nothing wrong with the use of such a closed language in appropriate arenas. However, with service users, the use of simple explanation and understandable language will often help to reduce the levels of anxiety experienced.

Equally, it is important not to ignore people, especially people who may become aggressive. In order to ensure that this impression is not being given, try to establish eye contact (without staring) at an early opportunity. Eye contact is a powerful communication tool. However, it must be remembered that some people from some ethnic backgrounds are not permitted to look into the eyes of another. Some people work on the basis that the eyes are the key to the soul, and in order to show respect eye contact is avoided. Some people show deference and respect by looking down towards the floor when they speak; while others will look over our shoulders. Eye contact is an important tool but it is influenced by ethnic, cultural and gender considerations.

The way we communicate is important and if we are perceived as arrogant, superior or patronising the potential for aggression is greatly enhanced. Yet so many times failure in the manner in which we communicate leads directly to increasing frustration in others.

9 Being kept waiting. *Never knowing when transport will arrive*

So there you are in that supermarket queue. You know, the one that stops when all the others have continued. So you decide to change queues, only to find that the one you get into then stops and the one you just left has now started again, and the person who was previously behind you is now getting served before you! Imagine the angst generated, yet in reality in such a situation we are only losing about five or ten seconds.

In social care we keep people waiting a lot longer than a few seconds, whether that is waiting for transport, to see a duty officer, to have breakfast, to be helped out of bed or a chair, and so on. Although it may not be possible to have a procedure for each situation, it is possible to consider such situations and our management of them. In society there are such procedures. In many hospital Accident and Emergency departments, for example, there is a time delay sign displayed: 'AVERAGE WAIT TO SEE A DOCTOR IS. . . .' On the Underground, the times of the trains are clearly displayed; and railway stations increasingly provide information screens detailing times and delays. As members of the public we may not like the information because it is often informing us of lengthy waiting times. At least, however, such information can often be empowering as it gives us some choice, even if it is only 'should I stay or should I go?'

ACTIVITY 2.10

In a group:

Identify and discuss the value of procedures within your work designed to help manage those situations where service users are kept waiting.

At an organisational level it may be possible to have a sign in some public buildings indicating the length of wait required before being seen by the duty officer. Time management techniques can be employed to ensure that time is being efficiently managed. The use of extra staff at key times or the installation of specialised equipment, such as that used for lifting and handling, are all ideas which, if employed, can help alleviate delays in service provision.

Individual care staff can also be instrumental in reducing the level of frustration generated, by being on time and keeping promises. Staff can further reduce the frustration level by appropriate communication. Be specific and say '*I'll see you in twenty minutes*', and not '*in a few minutes*'. A few minutes to the service user could mean two or three; to you it could mean twenty or thirty. Do not say '*I'll see you later*' say '*I'll see you at four*'. Then arrive five minutes early and the perception of efficiency is created. Be wary, however – arriving twenty minutes early can produce the impression of being spied upon!

I know it is not always possible to arrive on time, because of other calls upon our service or even transport problems. If we do keep people waiting it becomes important to have another way to help manage some of the angst generated.

Reconsidering the previous example of the supermarket queue, what is the one thing the cashier could do or say to reduce some of the angst in the waiting customer? Often the answer is either SMILE AND BE PLEASANT or say SORRY.

Do not smile in the face of aggression as this will often be perceived as a smirk (see Chapter 5: Part A).

The use of the word 'sorry' can be influential but take care not to overuse it, especially within British society where the word tends to be overused. It must also be used with meaning and therefore feeling, so if it is not your fault you do not need to apologise, yet you can still make use of the word: '*I'm sorry you're so distressed, stop shouting, sit down and tell me about it*' (be careful about delivery which should be gentle and free-flowing). Or, if it is your fault: '*I'm sorry I kept you waiting.*' Then try not to use the word more than three times, as it then is often not perceived as genuine but merely a manipulative tool employed to attempt to stop behaviour.

10 Inefficiency. *Staff not doing what they say they will do*

Broken promises can be devastating, especially within situations where the person on the receiving end has a low self-image, feels inferior, or by circumstance is forced to rely upon others. Yet they regularly occur, as we promise 'someone will phone you back' and it does not happen, or 'I'll see you tomorrow' and we forget or become involved in other more pressing matters. Many promises made to children who come into the care of the agency are broken, leading to disaffective and hostile behaviour. Wherever possible maintain a promise. It is effectively a contract between you and the person concerned.

The impression of inefficiency can be caused by thoughtlessness. Take for example the situation where two shop assistants are talking together while you wander aimlessly around the store politely waiting for them to finish before they give you due attention. How many times do similar situations occur within your workplace? Situations where, for example, the care workers share a story or joke while giving a bed-bath or helping someone to eat; where the telephone dominates and is answered without apology during an information exchange; or even where the worker, unaware of significant changes in the service user's life, is tunelessly, happily whistling.

Inefficiency can be created by the introduction of new technology that is inadequate, or because staff are not properly trained to use it: 'Sorry, the computer's down.' Sometimes it may be due to an inability or unwillingness to accept responsibility: 'It's nothing to do with me.' While on other occasions it is created by under-staffing, which often leads to a lowering of staff morale and motivation.

ACTIVITY 2.11

Individually or in a group, identify:

Those areas in my work which appear inefficient are . . .
What are the causes for this?
What solutions do you propose?

Whatever the cause, the perception of inefficiency needs to be addressed as a core issue. If it is permitted to be maintained it helps to confirm the negative image of social care currently held by many in society.

If the elements identified in this chapter are some of the causes of aggression, IS THERE ANYTHING YOU CAN DO IN YOUR WORK STYLE, WORK PRACTICE OR YOUR WORK ENVIRONMENT to reduce the potential for these occurring?

KEY POINTS

By now you should be aware of some of the theories regarding aggression. You will have considered these theories and their relevance to your workplace. You will also have identified some of the causes of aggression which may be taking place around you and concerning your service users. Finally you will have identified some ways of reducing a number of those causes.

REFERENCES

1 Data Protection Act 1984. The Stationery Office.
2 A Protocol for Hampshire, Portsmouth, Southampton and the Isle of Wight: 'Potentially Dangerous Offenders'. Operational from 1 October 1998 to 30 September 2000. This protocol was developed and agreed by the Chief Officer's Group of Hampshire and the Isle of Wight, which comprises the Chief Constable, heads of local authorities, health agencies and other criminal justice agencies. This protocol relates to protection of the public from serious harm. It provides for an integrated, accountable approach to public protection and the sharing of appropriate information to allow for this.
3 NISW Briefing Number 26: 'Violence against social care workers': NISW, 5 Tavistock Place, London WC1H 9SN.

KEY READING

Archer, J. and Browne, K. (1989) *Human Aggression*. Routledge.
Berkowitz, L. (1993) *Aggression*. University of Wisconsin, Madison.
Coggans, N. (1995) *The Facts about Alcohol, Aggression and Adolescence*. Cassell.
Green, R. G. (1990) *Human Aggression*. Open University Press.
Kirsta, A. (1994) *Deadlier than the Male: Violence and Aggression in Women*. Fontana.
Lorenz, K. (1966) *On Aggression*. Methuen.
Storr, A. (1968) *Human Aggression*. Penguin.
Storr, A. (1991) *Human Destructiveness*. Routledge & Kegan Paul.

CHAPTER 3

ASSESSING RISK

Levels of violence can be reduced by assessing the risks staff are experiencing and wherever possible taking action or establishing processes to either eliminate or control those risks. The assessment of risk, whether around individual personal safety or the safety of staff for whom you may be responsible, need not be off-putting. It should not be reliant on completing yet another form within a form-filled system!

To be effective a risk assessment needs to be based upon an emerging body of knowledge and awareness. Within this, the risk assessment form is used as a device complementing and not dominating the process.

It need not be complicated to complete an assessment of risk – after all, making ongoing assessments is an existing part of the work of most social care staff. The focus of this assessment, however, requires a change in thinking. In this process the focus lies in assessing the risk to ourselves and those responsible to us, whereas usually social care staff focus on the needs of and risks to the service user.

OBJECTIVES

This chapter will:

- Identify the legal situation regarding personal safety, and in particular will consider health and safety legislation.

- Aid in the assessment process by highlighting those factors that indicate the potential for a higher level of risk as they relate to: (a) the service user (b) the environment and (c) staff.

- Realistically consider what may be done to reduce the risk of violence to staff.

- Provide an example of a formal risk assessment, giving those charged with the responsibility for completing risk assessments a useful outline.

WHAT THE LAW REQUIRES

There are six main pieces of health and safety law that are relevant to violence at work in England and Wales. These are:

- **The Health and Safety at Work Act 1974**
  Employers have a legal duty under this Act to ensure, so far as is reasonably practicable, the health, safety and welfare at work of their employees.
  Employees have an obligation also to ensure their own health, safety and welfare *and* that of their colleagues.

- **The Management of the Health and Safety at Work Regulations 1992 and 1999**
  Employers must:
  - assess the risks to the employees and identify ways to reduce those risks
  - where there are five or more employees, record the important findings of the risk assessment
  - implement the measures identified as necessary by that risk assessment
  - make arrangements for planning, organising, controlling, monitoring and reviewing health and safety measures
  - appoint competent people to do this
  - provide information and training for staff
  - work with other employers sharing the same workplace
  - complete risk assessments for particular employees, especially pregnant women and young employees

  The risks covered should, where appropriate, include the need to protect employees from exposure to reasonably foreseeable violence.

- **The Reporting of Injuries, Diseases and Dangerous Occurrences Regulations 1995 (RIDDOR)**
  Employers must notify their enforcing authority in the event of an accident at work to any employee, resulting in death, major injury, or incapacity for normal work for three or more days. This includes any act of non-consensual physical violence done to a person at work.

- **Safety Representatives and Safety Committees Regulations 1997 (a)**

- **The Health and Safety (Consultation with Employees) Regulations 1996 (b)**
  Employers must inform and consult with employees in good time on matters relating to their health and safety. Employee representatives, either appointed by recognised trade unions under (a) or elected under (b), may make representations to their employer on matters affecting the health and safety of those they represent.

Additional requirements

The employer's liability at Common Law to protect employees and others against personal injury is part of the general law of negligence. To establish a claim for negligence, generally within three years of the date of the incident, the onus of proof is on the employee who must show that:

1   The employer owed the employee a duty of reasonable care in terms of the provision of a safe system of work, a safe place of work and safe plant and appliances.
2   The employer was in breach of that duty.
3   As a result the employee suffered damages.

An employer who is liable to an employee for damages will have a claim for some reimbursement against another party liable for the same damages, e.g. a negligent employee for whom the employer is vicariously liable.

Contributory negligence, which is the extent to which the injured party failed to take reasonable care of him/herself as to constitute one of the direct causes of the incident, may be pleaded as a defence by the employer.

The employer is likely to be regarded as negligent only if he or she does not take steps to eliminate a risk that he or she knows or ought to know is a real risk.[1]

Penalties for failure to comply with health and safety law

Magistrates can impose fines of up to £40,000 for offences under Sections 2–6 (general duties) of the Health and Safety at Work Act, or for failure to comply with Improvement and Prohibition notices. Individuals can be fined up to £5,000 for failure to take action to prevent an incident of violence to staff from occurring if they knew or 'ought to have known' it would occur. Additionally individuals can face imprisonment of up to two years if they fail to comply with the requirements of health and safety law.

A DEFINITION OF VIOLENCE

The Health and Safety Executive, the official body that polices the health and safety legislation in England, defines work-related violence as:

> any incident in which a person is abused, threatened or assaulted in circumstances relating to their work.

This is an important definition as it recognises two key elements:

1   Violence is not purely a physical assault. Verbal abuse, threatening or intimidatory behaviour and threats are all considered as violence.
2   The incident may occur outside of normal office hours or even away from the work environment, yet if it originates from 'circumstances related to their work' the employer has a responsibility. An example requiring the employer to complete a risk assessment may involve a situation where the employee is living next door to a service user who bears a grudge against the employee for a decision taken while at work.

Legislation is one thing but in reality . . .

All too frequently risk assessments of the potential for violence towards staff are not completed. Even more worrying is that those people whose jobs are not risk-assessed are invariably those who feel less able to request a risk assessment or complain if one is not done. This is often because of their lowly position within the departmental structure. Yet frequently it is this group of staff who are most at risk.

SCENARIO

Lesley, a domiciliary care assistant – 'We're home helps really, but we're called domiciliary care staff because it sounds more professional I suppose' – *was asked to provide emergency cover over the weekend for a man about whom she had little information.* 'I was told he was 74 and that his wife had been admitted to hospital earlier that day. There were no relatives around and he had very little food in the house, so could I go in and get him some food and if necessary make him a meal.'

Apparently this is not an infrequent occurrence. 'It's not unusual, we get requests like this all the time. It's my job to go in if the duty social worker needs someone.'

Had a risk assessment been carried out on the situation? 'Well, if you mean had he been seen by anyone, no. The duty social worker was contacted over the 'phone by the doctor and he'd 'phoned me. That's the way it works. They get the information and pass it on to us.'

You say 'us' – does that mean you work in pairs? 'Oh no. We're on our own mostly, but we're told we can request a colleague to go along if we are worried. I usually ask my husband to go with me, especially if it's late at night. He waits in the car outside. Well you don't like imposing on colleagues, not really.'

On this occasion did you have your husband with you? 'No. It didn't seem at all worrying. We get requests like this all the time and it was still quite early by the time I was able to attend. It was about six and although the local shops would be closing the supermarket was still open so I wasn't that worried. It was a bit of a shock though when the old man, who had at first very pleasantly invited me in, slammed the bolt shut on the door and started ranting at me about being late and keeping him waiting all day! Well, I had no idea you see. I was fitting him in to the end of my schedule. Apparently he had been told by his doctor that morning to expect somebody around "soon" but no one had told me that. He just carried on saying I couldn't treat him like rubbish and other stuff like that for I don't know how long. I was really scared. I know he was an old man but he was a lot bigger than me and he was standing in front of the front door. I said I'd better leave if he wasn't going to calm down but that just made him even worse.

I'd had enough and eventually I lost my temper and shouted back at him. Well that shocked him I suppose. I know we're not supposed to lose our temper with the clients but it just happened. I said if he wanted me to get him some food he'd better shut up and stop shouting. And you know what, he did. Well, I got a list from him and left. When I phoned the duty social worker to explain what had happened he said not to let it worry me. Just to get him the shopping making sure there was some fresh bread, and just leave it, not to bother doing any cooking. But if I could make him a few sandwiches to last him today and tomorrow.

> I was feeling a little shaky really but felt like a bit of a fool after speaking to the duty social worker. I didn't want to go back, not really, but like he said we couldn't leave the old man with nothing to eat.
>
> I was really anxious when I knocked on the door to go back in but the old man must have known he had gone too far before and he was as good as gold.'

ACTIVITY 3.1

Individually or in a group, identify:

1 The risk factors in this scenario.

2 List what could have been done to reduce the potential risk.

WHAT ELEMENTS MAKE UP A RISK ASSESSMENT?

There were a number of initial indicators in the above scenario which should have alerted both the duty social worker and the domiciliary worker to the potential for violence. Yet they were either not considered, or, if considered, an assessment had been made that the risk towards the domiciliary worker was low. The former is forgivable, the latter is not. Unfortunately all too frequently we put the needs of the client first, often ignoring the risk to ourselves, yet history does repeat itself and we can learn from the past.

Following situations of violence to staff it is often possible to identify similarities occurring within those situations. Identification of these similarities gives workers the opportunity of reducing future risk by taking them into account.

These similarities invariably involve at least three elements:

* the service user
* the environment
* the staff member(s)

ACTIVITY 3.2

In order to identify if there are any similarities relating to the above within your work:

PART 1
In a group of three participants, nominate one person to tell of the events leading up to a situation where they faced or witnessed aggression, nominate one person to make notes, and one person to ask questions to help the story unfold.

Start by describing the actual event and then work back to consider the immediate circumstances occurring prior to the incident. Identify any potential TRIGGERS which may have contributed to the incident (include any significant people involved, their age, gender, level of experience, etc.).

Next identify in particular any significant HISTORY in the service user, either known at the time or identified subsequently.

PART 2
Once all three situations have been considered:

As a group identify ANY SIMILARITIES within the three situations outlined.

Typical similarities include:

The service user

1   mental illness and the mythology
2   history of violent or aggressive behaviour
3   the behaviour itself
4   appearance
5   alcohol/drugs
6   threats
7   change
8   frustration
9   lack of alternatives
10   possessions
11   removal of/power over liberty
12   relationship
13   recently expressed aggression
14   service user is unknown or no information

1 Mental illness and the mythology

There is a myth around mental health which suggests an association between mental illness and violence. In fact mental illness incorporates an enormous range of a variety of states including depression, anxiety disorders leading to fear and phobias, schizophrenia, effective psychosis, dementia, memory loss, paranoia, psychotic and delusional states, and so on. Each of these categories will also have sub-categories. It must be borne in mind, therefore, that within society a great many people will be getting on with their lives while also having been labelled as 'mentally ill'. The vast majority of these individuals are likely to be non-violent. This has been identified in research. One study completed in the USA, regarding the link between mental illness and violence, identified:

(a)   The vast majority of people with mental illnesses are not violent, nor are they criminals.

(b)   Mental illness is not a good indicator of violence – substance abuse, age and gender are more reliable predictors.
(c)   Persons with mental illnesses are more likely to be victims of crime.[2]

Paradoxically, in social care the myth may have some basis in fact. Of the eight social care staff who have died at the hands of service users since 1984, four were murdered by service users who were mentally unwell. While it must be remembered that there were other contributory factors within each of these situations, a safety-first approach must dictate the use of two workers when dealing with mentally ill people who are deemed to be dangerous, either to themselves or to another person, especially in circumstances requiring compulsory admission to a hospital. Invariably this does not happen, and too frequently the Approved Social Worker is left alone, waiting for the arrival of the ambulance, with someone of 'diminished responsibility', as the other professionals pull out.

    The general rule for dealing with a person who is mentally unwell is: treat them as you would a normal person. However, if the person is paranoid and you are becoming or have become the subject of that paranoia, be careful. Secondly, if the person is hallucinating and/or deluded *and* the hallucinations or delusions are negative and hostile, be on guard. Furthermore if the person then begins to direct the hostility towards elements associated with you or your job, even beginning to identify you as a representation of those elements, then at that stage, if not before, common sense dictates you take appropriate action to manage the situation. Often it becomes appropriate to leave.

2 History of violent or aggressive behaviour

All too frequently it has been revealed that the person who was aggressive had a history of being so. One tragic case illustrating this was that of the social worker Isobel Schwartz, murdered by a service user who had previously attacked her. Isobel remained involved with her client because, according to her father, '*Isobel had established a relationship*'.[3] Unfortunately this situation has been repeated on many occasions – thankfully not with the same consequences. Care workers try their best to establish a relationship with the client and will attempt to maintain it, often irrespective of physical assault. Within too many homes for older people, care workers put up with being hit because '*it's only her way*' and '*she doesn't mean it really*' or '*when he's better he's a lovely man*'.

    The previous violence need not have been directed at you – it might have been aimed at another professional or a colleague. It may have even been directed at a person whom you have now come to represent. If the person has been violent in the past this must be considered as evidence for potential violence in the future.

3 The behaviour itself

Watch for behaviour at three levels:

- behaviour that is escalating
- behaviour that is out of the 'norm' for the person concerned
- behaviour that is unpredictable

Behaviour that is escalating

Escalating behaviour may take place immediately before the incident. The person may begin to show minor signs of agitation which slowly or even rapidly increase. Be alert for increased repetitive body movement ranging from tapping, strumming of fingers, to head nodding and body rocking. Speech levels may rise along with a quicker delivery. Tonal changes may take place and speech may become more shrill. Pacing may also occur, either as a continuation of this process or in its own right.

Escalation may also have been taking place over a long period of time – for example, a few months ago complaints may have been made which went ignored. Over time the complaints become more demonstrative and pronounced until finally the person explodes.

Behaviour that is out of the 'norm' for the person

Sometimes a person who is usually active can become very still. Sometimes the behaviour may become bizarre, with florid arm movements, for example. Sometimes it will be more subtle, almost imperceptible – an act or action that you know instinctively is not right. In these situations act upon instinct and take action to avert any possible aggression. Leave and discuss it with another professional.

Behaviour that is unpredictable

The one thing I will predict about unpredictable behaviour is that it will be unpredictable in the future! If behaviour has been unpredictable in the past we must take action to ensure safety in the future.

4 Appearance

People have a right to wear what they want to wear and it would be wrong to make an assumption associating dress-sense and violence. However, appearance can be an indication of mood and can even forewarn of violence. Some people associate violence with uniforms. With some people, however, it does not have to be the whole uniform. Some people associate violence with items of dress, insignia, badges or jewellery. If you are dealing with a person who begins to wear an item that signifies violence – and it could be a badge, a bandana, or a pair of gloves – be careful. It could simply be a fashion statement. It may, however, be a depersonalising process for the wearer, giving them the power vested within the representation of the image to violate you.

Other changes in appearance may be more easily identified. Physiological changes around the face, head and neck occur within many people who are becoming aggressive (see Figure 3.1).

Within some states of mental illness some people have been known to dress in a manner that gives an indication of mood. Some people have been known to wear bright, even garish, colours as an indication of their aggressive feelings.

Watch in particular for:

- a regular pronounced pulse in a vein in the forehead and/or at the side of the neck. Sometimes a regular pulse beneath one eye is apparent
- a colour change beneath the chin or in the whole face as the blood pressure changes (this could be lighter, darker or redder and is usually more visible in people with lighter skin colouring)
- a fixed eye stare with the eyelids coming closer together or even further apart
- the nostrils flaring as the person breathes rapidly and shallowly
- the mouth pulled tight with the teeth clenched

Figure 3.1 Aggression and physiological changes

Be alert for service users who have begun to let themselves go. It may simply be that they can no longer physiologically manage to maintain appearance because of illness, inability or increased frailty. If not, work on the basis that if they cannot care for themselves it will be harder for them to care about you, and subsequently therefore easier for them to damage you.

5 Alcohol/drugs

Alcohol and drugs are a high predictive factor that violence may occur. Be aware that often we are not dealing with the person we know. We are dealing with a product of what they have taken, and frequently the person will return the following day to apologise for their actions. Be careful of changes in prescribed medication which can result in a readjustment of behaviour. Some drugs are known to change behaviour. Be careful of people who are reducing, or coming off, medication. It can often lead to irritability and/or the expression of sudden explosive flashes of aggression.

Service users taking unprescribed drugs may not necessarily be violent in their behaviour. However, there is often a lot of associated violence within the user's life. Be careful if the user is changing or stopping their drug, in particular where this is not instigated directly by the user, and, even where it is, be on your guard for aggressive outbursts.

Alcohol is a drug. It is both a stimulant and a depressant and even though many of us enjoy a 'social drink' the same rules must apply. Alcohol is a disinhibitor – it allows individuals to do things they would not normally do, and that includes being aggressive. Be careful, therefore, of people who are changing their intake either by volume or type.

Do you have a workplace policy regarding alcohol?

6 Threats

Take threats seriously and act on them appropriately.

People use language to communicate and within aggression there are five common forms of language used. (See Figure 3.2.)[4]

TYPE	EXAMPLES	PURPOSE
Depersonalising language	you lot/ you staff/ you officials . . . you people	To perceive an OBJECT and not a human being
Degrading language	racist/sexist/ageist/ homophobic/personal comments	To perceive a person as of LESS WORTH/VALUE
Repetitive language	speech increases in speed or volume/word or phrase repeated	A WINDING-UP process
Emotional content	Sharp, short delivery (cultural differences mean this area is open to misinterpretation)	COVERT MESSAGE of inner feelings
Threats	To you/themselves/another or to the air	OVERT STATEMENT of action likely to follow and a PROCESS whereby the person is SOCIALISING themselves into the idea that they can carry out the act

Figure 3.2 Aggression and language use

A threat may be **verbal** – 'I'll do you', 'I know where your children go to school', etc. Or it may be **non-verbal** and identified as brooding and intimidatory, where the person may have intermittent eye contact or even a fixed stare, maybe with an associated almost imperceptible head nodding; or it may be **written**. Take written threats more seriously as they take time and energy to complete and demonstrate a commitment to act.

7 Change

We are an odd species in that in many ways we are constantly changing. Sometimes we change house, job, career direction, county, environment, relationship and so on. We are potentially therefore accustomed to change. However, change that is imposed is often reacted to negatively and this can show itself in the form of aggression. Imposed changes could include a change in status or ability or a change in medication. It could also be bereavement or loss, and it could be something as simple as a change of care worker.

8 Frustration

The day-to-day frustrations of which we are all aware, yet which still remain, are often the most infuriating. For service users, being told nothing can be done, knowing something can be, and not being listened to, are the most common ways care staff create frustration. Taking over and doing the task because of a lack of time, or patience, is another. Being lied to, talked about, laughed at, made to feel inferior, useless and, even worse, a burden are all other ways of increasing levels of frustration.

ACTIVITY 3.3

Individually or with your colleagues:

Identify those elements within your workplace that create feelings of frustration:

(a) within you

(b) within your service users

Next, discuss what can be done to eliminate or reduce these elements.

---

9 Lack of alternatives

Always give alternatives. If there is no alternative, if you are the one perceived as ultimately giving the negative decision, then effectively the person has nothing more to lose and the potential for an aggressive act is increased. Do not give ultimatums. Try to give choice and options, even if the only other option is to enable the service user to complain about the lack of alternatives to someone in power – a local councillor or Member of Parliament.

Sometimes the unavailability of alternatives lies within the service user who has been expressing him/herself in an aggressive manner for many years simply because he/she knows no other way. A powerful way of enabling some service users to both achieve their goals and feel good about themselves, thereby improving self-esteem, is to teach alternative ways to express anger and frustration (see Chapter 9).

10 Possessions

Lots of people invest significant amounts of value in items that to other people would be worthless. It could be that the item holds sentimental worth, intrinsic value not known to others, or the item could be the element that connects the individual to a memory or even to reality. It could be the only thing in the universe actually belonging to the individual concerned. Imagine one thing that is truly yours, that which you value above all else. Now imagine that someone were to come and attempt to take that thing from you. How would you feel, and what would you do to stop that from taking place?

The item concerned could be as insignificant as the plastic bag in which the child carried their belongings on admission into residential care; it could be a cup, a chair, a plate, a comb. Within residential care how many times do we hear the cry 'She's sitting in my chair!', when in reality we all know that the chair actually belongs to the home?

The remnants of a security blanket are kept by many and defended by some. It could be the bottle belonging to the drunken person, a last photograph, or a piece of paper with a scrawled note from a relative or friend. Some people also regard their children as their possessions. Some their animals.

Do not interfere with a person's possessions without asking permission. Wherever possible, ask the person to move them or, in the case of the drunk with the bottle, to put it down.

If you are ever faced with having to remove possessions from a service user always consider this a time of potential high risk and take appropriate precautions.

11 Removal of/power over liberty

This is a high predictive factor for potential aggression. Within child and family work it has long been recognised that taking a child into care against his/her will is fraught with dangers. In such circumstances the worker will always be accompanied. Within the other social care areas, the concept of there being two workers to, for example, remove a man suffering from dementia from home for placement within a residential setting, or to remove the liberty of a person deemed mentally unwell, is still, in too many agencies, unclear. All too frequently, social care staff take people into a care establishment unaccompanied and often in their own cars. Alternatively, the care worker may find themselves alone with the person for hours, awaiting the arrival of the ambulance, or even accompanying the person to mental hospital, or a care home – sitting in the back of an ambulance, without the presence of another professional, but with the person who perceives them as being responsible for taking away their liberty.

12 Relationship

Most forms of violence take place within an established relationship. Within social care, recent research has identified that the person most likely to be at risk of violence is the female worker (possibly because there are more female care workers), who is younger (potentially therefore less experienced), *and* commonly after about six months of being involved with the service user.[5]

13 Recently expressed aggression

How many times have you managed a situation of aggression only to have it flare up again perhaps only minutes later? In many instances it takes the aggressor a long time to actually get themselves into a state whereby they can perform the act of aggression. Equally it takes the aggressor a long time before their emotional level is once again reduced. Often the energy is there just below the surface waiting to re-emerge. An overall average length of time for the dissipation of the feelings is about ninety minutes.

However, within some individuals it can be a lot longer. If you have dealt with an aggressive incident, therefore, do not assume it is now over – be alert to the potential for it to resurface. Take affirmative action, perhaps ensuring the aggressor is occupied in a constructive task which will help them to let the anger go, or even removing yourself and others.

14 Service user is unknown

Some agencies have taken the position that if the person is not known to them two staff will be initially involved. This is irrespective of the service user's age, gender or situation, which may be the only known facts. It is a common-sense, safety-first approach which helps increase staff safety. In reality the majority of people who are dealt with for the first time are going to be non-violent. As the Arabic proverb states, however, 'Trust in Allah but always tie up your camel at night!' After all, Mr Kipper* is still out there.

The environment

Sometimes staff work in areas that are potentially dangerous. This may be an estate which has a high incidence of drug-related crime, an area reputed for gang activity, an area where muggings are frequent, or one where other professionals such as fire, health or postal workers have been 'targeted'. Alternatively, the environment may be an isolated interview room at the end of a long deserted corridor. The environment may include lonely walkways, poorly lit car-parking areas, and empty buildings where at the end of the day one worker is left alone to lock up.

Alternatively the environment could be the empty open countryside.

CASE STUDY

Tony was asked to do a follow-up visit on a woman who had been discharged from hospital where she had been treated for depression. Her husband farmed land on Todmorden moor. I had seen her a few times in hospital and didn't think much about it really. It was nearly Christmas and we'd collected some toys which I knew she would like for the kids.

It took some finding. I had to park my car at the end of a narrow lane and climbed over the stile. Then after following the path across a field it started to snow. I thought I wasn't really dressed for this! But trudged on knowing that as I'd come this far it would be stupid not to carry on. Anyway I was really relieved to see the farmhouse, but a bit disturbed when the young woman came to the door in her dressing gown. In my mind I imagined a scene where her husband

---

* 'Mr Kipper' was the last appointment for Suzy Lamplugh, the estate agent who has been missing since 1986.

would come back and find us alone together. I felt really vulnerable. I pushed the toys at her and bumbled something about not being able to stay because it was getting late and I left. Even now thinking about it I think to myself how stupid I was. She could have said anything and my career would have been ruined. I even imagined that because he was a farmer he could quite easily have had a gun and then who knows? I'll never do it again. Not visiting someone that isolated by myself. You learn, don't you?

Although this happened some years ago, even today individual members of staff are alone and vulnerable in isolated parts of the country.

ACTIVITY 3.4

Individually or with your colleagues:

Identify those situations in your work in which you have been alone and where you have felt vulnerable.

Other environmental factors to consider occur within the facilities provided for service users. Poor surroundings, shoddy furnishings, enclosed spaces, inadequate lighting, lack of facilities, run-down waiting areas – all give the impression of our lack of worth for the service user and all increase the possibility of aggression.

The staff member

In order for an assessment of risk to be complete, it is essential to consider the individual skills, abilities, circumstances and attitudes of staff members who are to be involved. This is invariably an ongoing process which should take place with staff supervision. Indeed many agencies have a 'Staff Supervision Policy' which covers both the frequency and content of supervision to aid the manager.

Not all staff have the skills to deal with conflict and sometimes additional training in this area may be required. Even then, some staff remain unable to manage and that must be recognised. Sometimes ability is influenced by ill-health, home or family life, excessive stress, or the million and more elements that make up human existence. Some of us are better able to manage situations in the morning, others function better later in the day and so on. Skills can be influenced and improved, abilities and circumstances can be changed, yet often attitudes are deeply embedded. Attitudinal change is one of the most difficult things to accomplish, and within social care four particular attitudes often increase the potential danger.

All too frequently following a violent incident it can be identified that the care worker felt RESPONSIBLE for either the service user or the circumstance facing the user. This feeling of responsibility, whilst commendable, is one that can put individuals at risk. It can create circumstances whereby the worker stays too long, visits too frequently, intervenes inappropriately, or even returns too readily to a situation where violence has taken place.

Secondly, the MACHO attitude is one still prevalent within some staff, though it is not as easily identified as perhaps the term indicates. It can be hidden within the culture of the working unit (see Chapter 1) and may be evidenced by individuals who praise an ability to 'cope' with violence while decrying as weak those who cannot. It can be based upon a desire to be perceived as capable, effective and strong and may be enmeshed within the British 'stiff upper lip' approach which suggests that if you cannot take it you should not be there.

Equally important is the LAISSEZ-FAIRE attitude leading to the blasé approach. This can feature within agencies where violence against staff is low, infrequent or not recent. It often exists within more experienced workers who, having been in social care for many years without incident, fail to take appropriate steps to safeguard themselves. It can be evidenced by the worker who, without leaving notification of his/her whereabouts with anyone, calls on their way home on a Friday evening to see a service user to discuss a difficult matter.

Additionally the UNCARING attitude, which is demonstrated in performance and is often derived from burnout or pressure of work, can create a desensitisation of the service user, leading in turn to an offhand, even offensive, manner.

ACTIVITY 3.5

In a group, identify:

1 Those attitudes that may create an aggressive reaction within the service user.

2 The attitude is demonstrated by . . .

Individual circumstances need consideration

Additional risk assessments are required for specific groups of workers, in particular pregnant women and young employees (HSE regulations 1999).

A recent research study carried out by the University of Hertfordshire indicated that female care staff experience more violence than male staff and report more incidents of sexual violence than their male counterparts.[6] This, however, could be due to the fact that female staff are disproportionately represented within social care.

In a study carried out by the National Institute for Social Work[7] it was identified that younger staff were more at risk of violence.

As well as age, gender and ethnicity must be considered. For example, it would not be appropriate to allocate a black worker to a known racist. Equally it would be inappropriate to allocate a white or black male worker to deal with an Asian Muslim female service user. The caste system still operating within some cultures may need to be considered before allocating a care worker, who may be from one caste, to a service user from a different caste.

RISK ASSESSMENT – THE FORMAT

A risk assessment format generally comprises five stages:

- Stage 1: IDENTIFY THE RISKS

  Discuss with staff who are involved. Take into account feelings of vulnerability and previous incidents. Establish a recording system in order to gather information (I have included a simple INCIDENT REPORT FORM outline at the end of Chapter 4 – see pp. 72–3).

- Stage 2: DECIDE WHO MAY BE HARMED AND HOW

  This may be one specific worker or a group of workers. The harm may be either physical or psychological.

- Stage 3: EVALUATE THE LEVEL OF RISK AS HIGH, MEDIUM OR LOW

  Make use of the information contained within this chapter to determine the potential risk level. Consider the information pertinent to:

  - the service user(s)
  - the staff member(s)
  - the environment(s)

  If the level of risk is determined as high, action is required to reduce the level; for medium risks controls should be put into place; and for a low level of risk no action is required.

- Stage 4: IDENTIFY THE MEASURES TAKEN TO REDUCE OR ELIMINATE THE RISK(S)

  This stage is often the most difficult for some agencies, as the argument of limited funds or resources is often used as a justification for not ensuring staff safety. The right for staff to be safe at work is enshrined in law, and stiff penalties can be imposed on individuals or agencies who fail in this. Furthermore the argument of 'no funds' is not accepted in law.

- Stage 5: REVIEW AND ASSESS THE EFFECTIVENESS OF THE MEASURES TAKEN

  As part of the assessment, you should decide when and how to undertake further reviews, which should, in any event, not be later than six months hence.

APPLYING THE MODEL

One area that I believe should always be risk-assessed is that of LONE WORKING, which within social care frequently occurs. Below is one outline which may be applied to situations in which one person is left to lock up a building at night and open a building in the morning.

- Stage 1: IDENTIFY THE RISKS

  RISK = One worker has been designated as part of her duties to lock up and open the building.

- Stage 2: DECIDE WHO MAY BE HARMED AND HOW

  WHO = Jane working alone on the premises at the beginning or end of the working day.

  HOW = Verbal abuse, including shouting, swearing, threats, personal comments and/or physical assault; resulting in fear, stress and/or physical injury.

- Stage 3: EVALUATE THE LEVEL OF RISK

  Yesterday at 8.15 a.m. Jane was stopped from entering the building by two men. Both wore masks. She was forced against the wall by the entrance and threatened. The threats concerned a specific situation involving one of the social work staff. She was unable to summon help, had not been provided with a personal alarm and felt more vulnerable in the dark – there is no outside lighting.

  Following the threats the assailants ran off. This was a very dangerous situation and one which, because of the increasingly confrontational nature of our work, is potentially highly likely to happen again.

- Stage 4: IDENTIFY THE MEASURES TAKEN

  Jane is currently off work due to this incident. Two workers locked up the building last night and arrangements have been made for two workers to open the building each morning. The police have agreed to drive by each morning until the case referred to has been heard in court.

  For the longer term:

  1 Policy of two workers opening and locking up will remain
  2 Possibility of outside lighting to be examined
  3 CCTV to be considered
  4 Regular meetings with the local police to be instigated

- Stage 5: REVIEW AND ASSESS

  A staff meeting has been arranged for this afternoon, where discussion will take place of the measures taken and proposals made. Other ideas will also be considered.

  This situation will be reviewed weekly until the outcome of the court hearing (referred to in the threat) is known.

  Other risk assessments are being completed and measures are being taken to ensure safety for those workers involved in the case.

KEY POINTS

This chapter has:

- ☐ Given you information about health and safety and other legislation applicable to work-places employing five or more staff.
- ☐ Identified the potential liability facing individual staff and their manager(s) who fail to comply with the legislation.

☐   Identified elements that make up a comprehensive assessment of risk, and considered some ideas to reduce those risks.

Finally it has:

☐   Provided an outline of a usable model of risk assessment, including an example of the format being used within a specific situation.

By now you should be aware of factors creating risks and have identified those elements present within your workplace. You will also have identified the ways in which these risks may be reduced, if not eliminated, in your work.

REFERENCES

1 East Sussex County Council policy statement.
2 *Violence in Homes and Communities. Prevention, Intervention and Treatment* (1999). National Mental Health Association. Editors: Thomas P. Gullotta and Sandra J. McElhaney. Sage.
3 *Social Workers at Risk*. Thames TV programme made in 1986.
4 Braithwaite, R. (1992) *Understanding Violence: Intervention and Prevention*. Radcliffe Professional Press.
5 White, C., 'Keeping violence in mind.' *Community Care*. 28 Oct.–3 Nov. 1999.
6 See 5 above.
7 'Violence against social care workers.' NISW Briefing Number 26. NISW, 5 Tavistock Place, London WC1H 9SN.

KEY READING

Health and Safety Executive (1998) *5 Steps to Risk Assessment* INDG163 (rev). HSE Books.
Health and Safety Executive (1998) *Working Alone in Safety* IND (G)73 (rev). HSE Books (single copies free).
Health and Safety Executive (1996) *Consulting Employees on Health and Safety: A Guide to the Law* INDG232. HSE Books (single copies free).
Health and Safety Executive website: www.hse.gov.uk
Suzy Lamplugh Trust. *Reducing the Risk: Action Against Aggression at Work*. The Suzy Lamplugh Trust.

The National Task Force on Violence Against Social Care Staff was established following the death of Jenny Morrison who was killed by a service user in November 1998. The website contains comprehensive information for employees and employers:
www.doh.gov.uk/violencetaskforce

CHAPTER 4

ORGANISATIONAL RESPONSES TO VIOLENCE TOWARDS STAFF

Organisations responsible for staff are also responsible for staff safety. Violence may be directed towards an individual or a group of workers. It may take place between service users. It may involve one or more perpetrators. Sometimes it may take place between one employee and another. Irrespective of its make-up, managing aggression requires more than the approach of simply relying upon individual staff to have appropriate skills (see Chapter 5). It requires the organisation to adopt and employ proactive measures aimed at reducing levels of violence towards staff. This chapter will examine some of those measures.

OBJECTIVES

By the end of this chapter you should:

- Understand the value of reporting and why under-reporting of violence occurs.

- Be aware of a number of proactive responses employed by some agencies as a means of reducing the potential for violence to staff.

- Have considered ideas that it may be appropriate to make use of within your workplace.

Additionally, the management of the situation following violence is one that many agencies currently fail to consider. As it is good practice that staff are supported following an incident, this chapter will also:

- Provide a model for supporting staff who have experienced violence at work.

At the end of the chapter Figure 4.1 is a simple outline of a document used to report violence at work.

UNDER-REPORTING

Under-reporting of violence occurs in many instances because of:

- no, or inadequate, definitions of violence used by organisations
- a non-supportive workplace culture which fails to encourage reporting (previously covered in Chapter 2)
- lack of awareness by staff concerning what they should record
- lack of clarity as to which report form to use
- not having the time to do it

It can be argued that any worker who is constantly facing a high bombardment of degrading language, derogatory words, racist or otherwise offensive personal comments may be more at risk of experiencing unhealthy stress levels than one who is not. A fundamental starting point for managing aggression at an organisational level, therefore, lies in the identification and recognition of the number and type of incidents of violence experienced by staff. Once the bombardment level is identified, the organisation can take steps to eliminate or reduce the risk. This is expected within current health and safety legislation:

> every employer shall provide his employees with comprehensive and relevant information on –
>
> (a) the risks to their health and safety identified by assessment;
> (b) the preventive and proactive measures [taken to reduce those risks].[1]

Organisations that fail to identify the levels of stress experienced by staff as a result of exposure to constant abuse do so at their own peril, as the compensation culture highlights. It is also good practice to encourage recording as a means of identifying trends, dangerous individuals or situations, triggers, and changes in practice required to better manage situations. Furthermore, accurate recording gives the organisation the opportunity to redirect resources and forward-plan appropriately.

Unfortunately, under-reporting of violence remains at a staggeringly high level; yet without a clear identification of the problem it becomes impossible to effectively manage that problem. Use the following activity as a way of identifying the level of violence within your work environment and the level of under-reporting that may be taking place.

ACTIVITY 4.1

In a group, using a flipchart:

1 Make a list of those words or behaviours which each of you have experienced in your work that have created damaging or hurtful effects physically or emotionally in you.[2]

2 Next draw a circle around each of these that you have officially reported on your agency's Incident Report Form.

3 Finally discuss your reasons for recording and/or not recording these incidents on the official form.

Many agencies remain unclear about those situations that need to be officially recorded. Some agencies fail to provide a recording process, while some offer a variety of Incident Report Forms to be used for different situations – e.g. accident, incident, near miss, verbal abuse and violence forms. Using different forms creates confusion in the employee and increases the difficulty of obtaining accurate information. Add to this the fact that many organisations still interpret 'violence' as a purely physical act – which actively discourages workers from reporting verbal and other forms of abuse – and reasons for under-reporting become clearer.

In September 1999, John Hutton, the then parliamentary Under-Secretary of State for Health, addressed a National Summit entitled 'Violence against social care staff', in which he gave the following definition:

> **what I mean by violence is incidents where workers are abused, threatened or assaulted in circumstances relating to their work, in ways which explicitly or implicitly challenge their safety, well-being or health.**

This definition once again identifies violence as more than a purely physical act and provides agencies with the opportunity to identify verbal and other forms of abuse as violence. Taking into account the law and the statement by the Under-Secretary of State, two obligations placed upon the organisation become clear. First, employers must identify WHAT constitutes VIOLENCE (within their organisation), and secondly, what they expect staff to officially record. This may not be a simple matter, however.

ACTIVITY 4.2

Think through, or in a work group, discuss the following:

1 If you are shouted at by an old man with senile dementia does that constitute 'violence'?

2 Would you fill in an Incident Report Form for such an event?

Many organisations are demonstrating good practice in this area by providing staff with clear guidance concerning what they should report. Staff are then enabled in that process by being provided with documentation and a procedure to achieve this.

Unfortunately, all too frequently the reporting document itself can create another barrier preventing adequate recording. The Incident Report Form can be up to five pages long in some agencies, and this will prove an insurmountable obstacle, especially when it comes to reporting incidents of verbal abuse, threats and threatening behaviours which may be a frequent occurrence in the particular workplace. If you are charged with the responsibility of drawing up such a form for your organisation, my advice is clear: keep it simple and make it user-friendly. At the end of this chapter I have provided an example of a simple one-page document used to report violence, with the reverse side being for completion by the line manager.

Besides the actual form used, on my training courses staff have frequently complained that they simply do not have the time to complete the paperwork following a violent episode. Nor is completing an Incident Report Form often considered a priority amongst other calls on time. Staff invariably put off completing the form until the end of a busy shift, at which point all they want to do is go home and put the incident behind them. If a comprehensive picture of levels of violence experienced by staff is ever to emerge, time and priority must be allocated by the organisation to ensure recording is achievable. One suggestion given on a recent training course was that one person be nominated in each workplace as the 'Violence person', with direct responsibility for ensuring that the Incident Report Form is completed, either by the individual concerned or by themselves. In this way incidents that may otherwise be 'lost' can be logged and identified. Another suggestion was that, instead of having yet another form to complete, the worker should have access to a telephone typing service (possibly a voice-activated computer) where he/she could telephone-in the incident for it to be officially recorded. This could both save time and encourage accurate recording. It was also felt that such a service might have the side-effect of being therapeutic for the victim. Although I remain unconvinced of the therapeutic value of such a notion, the idea of reducing the form-filling function is appealing.

PROACTIVE APPROACHES

Whilst increasing the number of recorded incidents is an important element in identifying and ultimately reducing the level of violence experienced by staff, there are a number of other steps that organisations can take on behalf of their staff.

In my training I often ask participants to identify any organisational responses to tackle violence that are employed by their agency.

ACTIVITY 4.3

In a group of four or five participants:

1 Identify those situations where you have witnessed or experienced violence at work.

2 Next state what was done to ensure it did not recur.

3 Finally, identify what initially could have been done by the organisation to reduce the potential for this violence occurring.

The following is a typical, though not exhaustive, list of proactive measures adopted by some organisations:

1   a violence policy
2   procedures in place involving lone working
3   an alcohol/drugs policy
4   practical safety ideas – i.e. personal equipment and office design
5   practising responding to alarms
6   reporting back or phoning-in for late or lengthy visits
7   a sign stating the rules regarding unacceptable behaviour
8   sanctions
9   clear rules about passing on information and confidentiality
10   use of codewords
11   staff training in methods of avoiding violence and managing aggression
12   post-incident support

1   A violence policy

Any policy document on violence to staff should be a clear and easy-to-use document. Some are so convoluted and protracted that they are worthless. Anyone charged with the responsibility for writing such a policy needs to avoid any woolly statements – staff need to know where they stand, what is expected of them, what they can and cannot do, and what they can expect from their agency. Be clear about these things. If you are unsure about any conflict between the goal of the agency to provide a service and the need to protect staff, use the basic premise:

ALL STAFF HAVE A RIGHT TO PERFORM THEIR JOB FREE FROM VIOLENCE OR THE FEAR OF VIOLENCE

Be aware that you do not have to reinvent the wheel – lots of organisations have very good policy statements simply waiting to be customised to meet the requirements of your organisation. Contact the personnel section or individual senior personnel within social care agencies close by. Many will be willing and even flattered to let you use their policy as a starting point for your own. Remember too that, just because the organisation has operated in a certain manner for many years, that does not mean the original approach was correct.

CASE STUDY

John, a residential social worker, was indoctrinated with the concept that the needs of the child were paramount. This was constantly reaffirmed to the point that within his working unit the staff began to accept the idea that 'a certain amount of violence had to be expected and tolerated'. John never considered his own needs and often went home exhausted and occasionally bruised. After a while the occasional bruise became almost a daily occurrence, which he accepted as a part of the job. He was, after all, he would argue, dealing with disturbed children who, he believed, had a right to be angry and the right to express that anger as aggression towards him and other staff. Finally, John was unable to take it any more. He began to dread going into work and on one morning two years ago chose not to. John has not worked in social care since.

ACTIVITY 4.4

In a group, discuss the above case study, answering the following:

1 Do you hold similar beliefs?

2 Do any of your colleagues hold similar beliefs?

3 What (if anything) is wrong with this approach?

A typical workplace policy on violence may well contain elements of the following:

- general statement of principles and values pertinent to the agency
- definition of violence
- health and safety and other pertinent legislation
- managerial responsibilities and obligations
- risk assessment (procedure and models)
- practical measures/responses
- reporting procedure
- post-event support (including debriefing, counselling, compensation, time off, etc.)

2 Procedures in place involving lone working

Not every lone working situation will create a high level of risk to staff safety. However, every lone working practice should be risk-assessed to ensure that the level of risk is low, or to identify measures that may be introduced to reduce the risk.

Particular attention should be paid to:

- opening and closing premises
- isolated working in a rambling building, or at the end of a long corridor, etc.
- solitary sleeping-in or night waking staff arrangements
- working in gardens with service user(s)
- accompanying service user(s) on shopping and other trips
- transporting service user(s) by car
- sole drivers of minibus/ambulance services
- visiting service user(s)

This area has been more fully covered in Chapter 3.

3 An alcohol/drugs policy

The following interview vividly demonstrates the value of an organisational response to violence generated by alcohol.

Julie is an Officer-in-Charge of a day centre for recovering mentally ill persons. Originally the centre was designated as a 'drop in', and operated an open door policy.

Julie: 'When I first arrived the policy of the centre was that throughout the day we never locked the front door. This meant that service users could arrive and simply walk in. The philosophy behind this being that this resource should be as accessible as possible to a disadvantaged and vulnerable group of people. Unfortunately, this meant that literally anybody could walk in any time of the day, and in the mid-afternoon in particular we had a problem with some service users arriving worse the wear from alcohol.'

Interviewer: 'What was the level of violence like within the centre at that time?'

Julie: 'High, very high. I think it was fair to describe us as almost under siege. Violent incidents were almost a daily occurrence. Fights were frequent amongst service users and staff were constantly having to confront dangerous situations. The staff felt unsafe. Stress levels were high. There was a lot of guilt and blame around. Guilt that we were letting the service users down and blame towards the system which created this environment. It's also fair to say that the staff group felt dis-empowered to bring about any change.'

Interviewer: 'So what did change it?'

Julie: 'We had some training in ways to manage aggression. During the training we clearly identified the major problems occurring in the centre in the early afternoon, and all the incidents talked about were alcohol-related. It was like a light going on. I know it sounds simple, but quite frankly it wasn't until we all were able to talk about the problem as a staff group that the solution appeared.'

Interviewer: 'What was the solution?'

Julie: 'Supervise entry into the building and refuse to allow anyone who had been drinking in.'

Interviewer: 'That sounds a little draconian. What about the rights of the service user to receive a service?'

Julie: 'But that was it you see. Beforehand service users came here because they had nowhere else to go and the majority of them were terrified of the fights. You could argue we were actually making their existence worse.'

Interviewer: 'So how did you achieve an alcohol-free centre?'

Julie: 'Once we had identified the extent of the problem it was relatively easy. I simply asked for a mortice lock (openable from the inside), an entry-phone and a perspex window fitted at the side of the door, so we could see who was coming in. Then we let everyone know that from the following Monday the centre would not operate an 'open door' policy, people would be let in and anyone who had been drinking would be refused entry. Then we put up signs in the building saying "No alcohol allowed on the premises", and that was it.'

Interviewer: 'What about the concept of user empowerment? Did you not ask what the service users felt about this change?'

Julie: 'Yes. All the attendees were involved in the decision and that really helped to swing it. But, to be frank, at the end of the day it came down to a management decision whether the agency would agree to a change in the use of the place and pay for the minor improvements required. With all the information about the incidents being mostly alcohol-related there was no argument and I was told almost by return memo to go ahead.'

Interviewer: 'And, now, what about the level of violent incidents?'

Julie: 'We haven't had an incident in over two years. And you know what, by and large, the same people are attending only now no one comes in drunk.'

ACTIVITY 4.5

Individually consider, or in a group, discuss:

Were the needs of the service users best served by this change, or have their 'freedoms' been denied?

Does your agency have a policy on alcohol?

The situation may become more complicated when visiting a service user within their own home. A person who is housebound, for example, may ask the worker to fetch them a bottle of wine or spirits. Should that be denied? My advice is to formulate a policy appropriate to the needs of your service and let your staff know what this is.

Similarly, if we are not to repeat the situation facing the 'Cambridge Two'[3] – where two voluntary workers were imprisoned for 'knowingly allowing' the use of drugs to take place within their presence – social care organisations must also ensure they have a policy on drugs, and staff must be informed what the policy is.

ACTIVITY 4.6

As a working group, identify within your work:

(a)   what elements a policy for alcohol should cover

(b)   a policy concerning drugs

---

4 Practical safety ideas

Many organisations issue **personal alarms** to their staff and this is good practice. Unfortunately not all will issue instructions regarding their use, and some staff remain unaware of their value. A personal alarm will not bring assistance. Once activated, it is designed to emit a high-frequency noise (screech) which it is hoped will distract any would-be assailant momentarily. This should be long enough to allow the victim to escape. Most personal alarms on the market are battery-operated and small enough to fit into a pocket or the palm of the hand. Some alarms also incorporate a flashing light which is marketed as a device for distracting assailants at night. The usual way of operating a personal alarm is by the removal of a pin, and the screech will not cease until the pin has been replaced. Gas-filled alarms, usually the same shape as and a little larger than a lipstick, are operated by depressing the top – the noise will continue while the pressure on the top is maintained.[4]

A personal alarm is valuable and can help distract a would-be assailant. However, they become valueless when carried in a bag or briefcase, or kept in the car, or even left forgotten in a desk drawer! Keep the alarm accessible, in the hand, in an outside pocket or attached to a belt. Generally, they should not be activated within an enclosed space as the noise level is so great with some that they could damage the eardrum.

Closed circuit TV (CCTV) is used by some organisations both inside and outside of buildings. It can prove a deterrent as its use in inner city and town areas has demonstrated, and need not be costly – some systems cost as little as a few hundred pounds. Many organisations have installed CCTV into specific interview rooms which are then used for situations where the potential for aggression has been identified. A particular deterrent used by some organisations is to tell the person being interviewed of the CCTV prior to the interview.

It is irresponsible of an organisation not to provide **emergency alarms** within offices where staff interview service users. Emergency alarms vary. Many emergency alarm systems produce a loud noise, either a bell ring or a siren. Silent alarms are also available – once activated they cause a light to flash on a monitor, so alerting another member of staff to the difficulty. Many alarms are fixed into the wall. Unfortunately all too frequently these are placed for convenience next to the light switch, when invariably they are needed elsewhere in the room. Portable silent alarms may be carried by the individual worker and can be more useful.

Mobile phones are often provided, especially for lone workers, and can help individuals to feel safer. There are, however, 'dead' zones where no signal is received by the mobile phone, and frequently the zone can be in the high-rise building being visited. They need to be tested in such areas to ensure a signal is received. In emergencies, rather than having to type in a complete telephone number of up to eight or more digits, it is possible to key-in a memory-retained telephone number, allowing the worker to simply press one button which sends a prearranged code signal to a colleague (see 'Use of code words', p. 67).

Incidentally, a **two-way radio system** is a less costly option for use within a small geographical area. These hand-held, battery-operated units are usually effective within a range of up to a few miles, and can be extremely useful in allowing staff to remain in contact with colleagues when working alone, or with a group of service users, in the grounds of an establishment or within a multi-storey block for example.

Perspex security screens, through which the service user can be seen, have been installed by some agencies in reception and other areas. I remain concerned about the use of such screens, which may be perceived as a barrier to good communication. Their use in interview room doors may be an advantage where service users have a known history of aggression, but the installation of such screens must be appropriate. I would always recommend any agency thinking of installing them to contact other organisations which have screens installed to discuss their value. CCTV remains a better option.

Office/room design is always an important consideration. Specifically consider having two entrances in opposite sides of the interview room, to reduce the potential for the worker to have their exit blocked. Where this is not possible, try to ensure equal accessibility to exits for both worker and user by rearranging the layout of seats, tables, etc. Think about rehanging interview-room doors – and other doors that may create an obstacle – so that they open outwards, allowing for a swifter exit. Secure furniture to the floor to prevent it being thrown (and secure it in a user-friendly manner). Avoid providing potential missiles such as heavy ashtrays. Ensure a 'safe area' for staff – coded locks can help in this process.

In residential and day-care units, pay particular attention to the items available to the service user, especially ensuring that all knives and tools are returned to a secure area or cupboard after use. Look around those environments open to, or used by, the public and identify any possible items that could be used as weapons and then make them safe.

ACTIVITY 4.7

Individually or in a group, identify:

(a) what devices would be useful in your work to help you to feel secure and how could these be used?

(b) what items could be used as 'weapons' in your workplace and what could be done to reduce the potential for the item being used?

---

5 Practising responding to alarms

So many times staff who attend my training have said that, although they do have emergency alarms in their building (these are usually ones that ring, or screech, loudly), they have no idea what to do should one go off! The commonly held view is that, should the alarm ring, all staff nearby should respond. If this is the case in your workplace, when everyone has rushed into the room where the alarm originates, what happens next? Who does what? This needs to be considered to allow staff to be clear about the procedure. Is, for example, one person nominated as the negotiator should a weapon be involved, or do you trust to luck that someone will say and do the right thing?

A silent alarm discreetly activated can allow a colleague to enter the interview with a spurious 'telephone call for you', thereby extracting the worker.

6 Reporting-back procedure

Frequently staff complete home visits either at the end of the day or even in the evening. Sometimes staff may spend the whole day visiting different service users. Such visits can take place without recourse to any contact with the office, maybe starting and finishing from the worker's own home without the worker having made colleagues aware of their whereabouts. Occasionally a cryptic clue may be left in an office diary: '*Visits – all day – not back*.' In order to protect staff in such situations it is essential that organisations adopt a report-back or a call-in procedure. This could either be in person or by telephone.

Some organisations have established a system whereby the worker leaves details of destination and probable length of involvement, as well as expected time of call-back. Should the call-back not be accomplished by an agreed time, the police are informed and action to trace the individual will commence. An example of such a system presently being employed is on the Isle of Wight, where council staff detail their movements and the tracing process is begun if the call/report-back procedure is not completed within the identified time.

What would you think about such a procedure being adopted in your work?

---

7 A sign stating the rules regarding unacceptable behaviour

Signs clearly indicating a negative outcome for bad behaviour are becoming common-place within some organisations:

> *Action will be taken against members of the public who assault staff* (London Underground)

> *No violence. No drugs* (various public houses)

> *If you are abusive or offensive to a member of staff or towards another member of the public you will be asked to leave and the police may be called* (various public houses)

> *No abusive language or behaviour* (East Sussex County Council)

Qualitative research completed in April 1999 on behalf of the Government's National Task Force on Violence Against Social Care Staff, found:

> At a more practical level, respondents suggested that having . . . **clearly displayed notices stating the ground rules for client behaviour and the consequences of bad behaviour** . . .would help considerably to prevent problems.[5]

See also 'The concept of zero tolerance' – Chapter 1, p. 15.

8 Sanctions

The use of a sign which states the rules for unacceptable behaviour can only work if the service user is educated into different ways of expressing anger (see Chapter 9) **and** if the organisation is prepared to take sanctions against perpetrators of violence (see Chapter 1). All too frequently the issue of sanctioning behaviour amongst service users is considered either distasteful or unprofessional, and arguments like '*we cannot further disadvantage the disadvantaged*', or '*they can't help it*', and even '*it would be bad for the profession*' are used. If a care worker did to a service user even a small proportion of the things that some service users do to them, action would, quite rightly, be taken. Yet all too often aggressive behaviour from a service user is ignored. The behaviour must be worked with and sometimes that means providing clear boundaries regarding behaviour, including the measures the organisation is prepared to take should that behaviour involve violence towards staff or another service user.

What sanctions do you use in your work to deal with violent or aggressive behaviour?

9 Clear rules about passing on information and confidentiality

Frequently information concerning the service user is not available to the care staff involved. A variety of arguments for this exist:

- information not received from another agency
- provided on a need-to-know basis only
- withheld in the interests of the service user
- confidential to another agency
- file gone missing
- it will arrive tomorrow

Staff safety comes before client confidentiality, and in those situations where the information is late in arriving, or not available, safety-first procedures must be considered. Furthermore it is good practice that information is available to all staff who are dealing with service users.

Are you always provided with the necessary information to ensure your safety?

10 Use of codewords

CASE STUDY

Susan called to do an assessment following supervision with her manager where they had discussed the possible risk of the client becoming aggressive. She wanted to call alone even though they had identified that the young woman had previously been aggressive towards other 'officials'. In hindsight it was a mistake but at the time it felt the right thing to do, mostly because Susan felt she knew the young woman and wanted to maintain her trust. The one thing Susan and her manager had agreed upon was that she would take a mobile phone and, as an afterthought, and a bit of a joke, she also agreed with her manager that if she encountered any problems she could always phone-in with a codeword. If she could not talk freely she could say something like 'I need the blue file', and that would mean 'Get me out of here!' They had both laughed.

It was two hours later when Susan phoned and used the code and her manager realised she was in danger. Unfortunately, at this stage no one had considered the next move – how to extricate Susan from the danger. The manager contacted the police who used armed personnel to secure the building and a negotiator to deal with the client. Susan was released some hours later.

ACTIVITY 4.8

In a group discuss:

1 Do you make use of codewords within your work?

2 What do you think about the value of codewords?

3 What can be learned from the above case study?

The use of codewords can never replace appropriate staffing, and sometimes working in pairs is imperative, as is rethinking the location of the interview. In those situations where there is a potentially high risk that violence may occur (see Chapter 3), wherever possible the client should be seen within the office or another 'safe' environment. Never become complacent, however – too many workers have been violated during 'routine' office interviews. Codewords have successfully been employed by reception staff, day-care and residential as well as domiciliary workers, in order to convey difficulty, where a less subtle approach would possibly escalate the danger.

11 Staff training in methods of avoiding violence and managing aggression

There are a lot of different trainers and training packages covering the subject of violence at work. The providers vary in their effectiveness and ultimate value to the individual and organisation. Always ask for and seek references. Do not accept unsubstantiated claims regarding the numbers of people stated to have received the particular package of training offered. External training in the subject is usually provided as a one- or two-day programme (excluding methods of holding, or restraining). The training could be provided on-site. However, training away from the workplace often allows staff to focus on the subject without becoming involved in the day-to-day work. The individual or organisation providing the training usually requires you to provide a venue and the equipment, such as overhead projectors, video playback units, flipcharts and paper.

Good training is specifically tailored to meet the needs of the organisation as well as the needs of the individual participants. Avoid providers who are reluctant to feed back issues arising from the training, especially where those issues are raised by participants.

Good practice for providing specific training in methods of physically intervening requires that this form of training is provided only after staff have been trained in avoidance, awareness, defusion and other interpersonal communication skills. A good training provider will not offer training in physical intervention methods in isolation, and caution must be applied if any trainer offers this form of training as a stand-alone package.

12 Post-incident support

Staff who face violence at work usually experience an emotional aftermath (see Chapter 8) and will often require help to overcome this. The help need not be more than a common-sense approach of providing appropriate 'support', but then what does this term 'support' actually mean?

In practice, support can often mean asking the person who has been subjected to violence what they want to happen next:

'Do you want to go home?'
'Shall I arrange cover for you or do you think you can cope?'

However, individuals who have been subjected to violence are not necessarily in the best frame of mind to be able to answer such questions.

ACTIVITY 4.9

With your colleagues discuss what you would want to happen next if you were:

(a) Slapped in the face by someone you were attempting to help?

(b) Spat at by the person?

(c) Held against the wall with a finger pointed in your face and told 'You are going to fucking die'?

(d) Hit over the head with a walking stick?

I believe the organisation owes staff a 'duty of care' and this includes ensuring that swift and appropriate responses are provided to any member of staff who has experienced violence. Not all staff will require the totality of the support model that I propose, but it should be made available to all staff.

After an incident of violence, the effects – which in some instances can be long-lasting – need to be considered, and the following model can be useful in allowing staff to feel supported and valued by the organisation. Basically there are three stages to this model.

Stage 1: The immediate elements (the first few hours)

At this stage the situation has only just occurred. Turmoil may be ensuing as other staff are becoming involved; the noise, energy and activity levels are high; and for the person who has been the subject of the incident the emotions can be complex and raw. The needs of this staff member are equally as important as those of the service user(s), yet all too frequently they are put aside as the perpetrator and other service users become the focus of attention.

The immediate needs of the worker subjected to violence include:

- Being taken to a safe place. This will usually be away from the perpetrator and may involve the use of a separate building. Additional staff will usually be required in order to work with the perpetrator and be available for the staff member.
- Medical intervention if necessary.
- Reassurance and simply being asked 'How are you?'
- Acknowledgement that the situation is being resolved.
- Arranging for their duties to be covered and information that this is being done.
- Being taken home and arrangements made regarding their own vehicle.
- Contacting a family member or partner, and organising practicalities like arranging to collect their children from school.
- Decisions being taken regarding police involvement, and action to remove the perpetrator or ensure the safety needs of other staff.
- Information concerning the action taken to ensure no recurrence (either at this time or later, if appropriate).

Stage 2: Short term (from the first few days up to the next few months)

The worker's short-term needs include:

- Contact being made – either a telephone call or a visit if the worker is at home, or if they have returned to work a specific time set aside in order to debrief. Remember, however, that debriefing is considered effective if done on a number of occasions over a period of time, and potentially could be more harmful if only done on a one-off basis (see Chapter 8).
- Receiving a sympathetic letter of support and acknowledgement that this has happened from a senior member of staff within the agency can help.
- Information regarding the outcome of the situation, including what has happened to the perpetrator; information about financial details such as sick leave, insurance and compensation; information about their rights and legal action and what happens next, including discussion regarding return to work or redeployment.
- Talking about the possibility of external counselling if appropriate. At this stage, often workers are asked 'Do you want counselling?' and the answer is invariably 'No'. Be aware that the statement 'I think it would be good if you saw someone. I can arrange it if you like' means the same, yet is likely to elicit a more positive response.

- Arranging the completion of the Incident Report Form and completing a sensitive investigation.
- Planning for the future to help the individual to regain some feeling of control.

Stage 3: Longer term (three months plus)

- Ensure that one person is identified as a contact point who will have the responsibility to stay in touch and update. This provides the worker with a focus and maintains consistency.
- Discuss the possible reintroduction into the workplace and how this may be achieved. This may be problematic, especially in those situations where the perpetrator is still around.
- Discuss compensation issues including duration of full pay.
- Provide information regarding Criminal Injuries Compensation.[6]
- Identify possible redeployment options with the staff member and discuss these as a positive option.
- Discuss the possibility of legal action: the possibility of action brought against the perpetrator by the worker, or even an action against the organisation. The latter may be important, especially if the worker is unlikely to return to work because of the injury. If this is difficult, help the worker identify appropriate individuals to contact, e.g. union representative or solicitor (some solicitors will provide a 'No Win/No Fee' service *but* do read the small print as sometimes the 'no fee' element refers only to court action – letters and telephone calls may not be included).
- Identify what the worker wants to happen next and discuss the feasibility of this.

ACTIVITY 4.10

In a group of four or five identify:

What would you want to happen if you were the subject of violence at work:

(a) if the situation had only just happened?

(b) if you were now at home 'off sick' following the violence?

KEY POINTS

☐   Organisations can take many proactive steps to ensure staff safety.

☐   A key element in managing aggression lies in the identification of the number of incidents of violence experienced by staff.

☐   Once violence is identified, proactive measures can be taken to help reduce violence towards staff.

☐   It is important that staff have a clear message about behaviour that is deemed unacceptable.

SIDE A   COMPLETION BY EMPLOYEE

INCIDENT REPORT FORM

1. EMPLOYEE   Employee's name:

Department: Age:

Normal place of work:

2. WHAT HAPPENED   Date of incident: Time:

Location of incident:

Please give a brief account of the incident, including any relevant events leading to it.

3. DETAILS OF ASSAILANT   4. DETAILS OF WITNESSES

Name: Name:
Address: Address:
Age: Age:
Male/female
Other details: Other details:

5. CONSEQUENCE

Were you: Was there:

Verbally abused   Yes/No   Damage to personal property:......................

Words used:...   ....

Subjected to antisocial behaviour   Damage to agency property:........................

(e.g. spitting)   Yes/No

Please describe:.......................................

Injured   Yes/No

How?

Signed: Dated:

SIDE B   COMPLETION BY LINE MANAGER

---

6. REPORTING DETAILS

Date reported: Time reported: Reported by:

7. POLICE INVOLVEMENT

Have the police been informed?   Yes/No

If yes, by whom?

Date: Time:

Outcome:

8. MEDICAL OR OTHER AID GIVEN

Did employee receive medical   Yes/No   Was employee debriefed?   Yes/No
treatment?

Details:

Was employee taken home?   Yes/No

Details:

9. INJURIES REPORTED   Physical   Yes/No   Emotional   Yes/No

Details:

10. IMMEDIATE ACTION TAKEN TO ENSURE NON-RECURRENCE

11. ONGOING PLAN (including risk assessment and risk reduction measures implemented
and review date):

Signed: Dated:

Figure 4.1 Incident Report Form

☐   It is equally important that staff know what behaviour is to be officially reported.

☐   An organisation that cares for its staff offers a demonstrative model which then allows for staff to care effectively for the service users.

☐   Fundamental aspects of staff care involve:

- ensuring a reporting procedure

- making time available to record incidents

- employing proactive measures to reduce the potential for violence

- providing post-event support for staff who have experienced violence at work.

REFERENCES

1   *The Management of the Health and Safety Regulations* (1999). The Stationery Office.
2   Association of Directors of Social Services (1987) *Guidelines and Recommendations to Employers on Violence against Employees in the Personal Social Services.*
3   'Workers in drugs case suffer zero tolerance.' News article. *Community Care.* 25 Nov.–1 Dec. 1999.
4   The independent consumer guide *Which?* magazine carried out a product test on personal alarms in December 1994. Further information may be obtained from: Which? Ltd, Consumers Association, 2 Marylebone Road, London NW1 4DF (website: www.which. net).
5   *A Safer Place: Combating Violence Against Social Care Staff.* Report of the Task Force and National Action Plan. Department of Health. Jan. 2001 (www.doh.gov.uk/violencetask-force).
6   Criminal Injuries Compensation is available to individuals who have been subjected to assault. Information and forms for application can be obtained from: Criminal Injuries Compensation Authority, Tay House, 300 Bath Street, Glasgow G2 4lN (Tel: 0141 331 2726).

KEY READING

Bibby, P. (1994) *Personal Safety for Social Workers.* Commissioned by the Suzy Lamplugh Trust. Arena.
Taylor, G. (1999) *Managing Conflict.* Directory of Social Change.

CHAPTER 5

MANAGING AGGRESSION

There are many ways to manage aggression and this chapter will identify some of the ways available to us all. One important factor cannot be overlooked, however – there are some behaviours that are unmanageable and no matter how skilled, knowledgeable or experienced you are, SOMETIMES NOTHING WORKS.

In situations where nothing works, it is important to leave. This chapter will also consider this option and the conflict that may exist between the need to ensure personal safety and the difficulty of achieving it, particularly when by leaving a situation other service users may be placed at risk.

For the most part, however, there are things that can be said or done to manage aggression, and these interpersonal skills can be learned by the majority of us.

OBJECTIVES

This chapter will identify:

PART A   The effective use of body language within aggression and its value in helping to:
(a)   not inflame a situation, and
(b)   de-escalate a difficult situation.

PART B   Assertiveness – a way to manage the more covert forms of aggression, where for example the worker may be the subject of negative criticism, made to feel inadequate, have their competence questioned, or made to feel uncomfortable and coerced into doing something.

PART C   Defusion techniques – words and/or actions we can all employ which can help manage those high levels of energy, to get them out of the way in order that we may continue to deal with the individual, or ensure personal safety.

> ▦ PART D Physical intervention as a means of managing aggressive behaviour, and we will consider some of the legal and moral issues pertinent in control and restraint.
>
> By the end of the chapter the reader will be aware of a variety of ways to manage difficult situations, difficult feelings and difficult behaviours; in short, the reader should be equipped to manage aggressive behaviour.

PART A

THE EFFECTIVE USE OF BODY LANGUAGE

Context

Body language is a non-verbal form of communication which occurs between individuals. It is clearly identified within the animal kingdom where it is less open to misinterpretation. In humans, body language varies, and in this section I will focus upon the meaning and interpretation of body language within aggression. In particular I will highlight the positive aspects of body language which may be employed by the worker to help de-escalate aggression. I also want to consider some of the processes involved which will influence many of us. Some of these processes will inadvertently bring about body language that can be perceived as negative and may require amending.

As about 70 per cent of all communication takes place at a non-verbal level it is extremely important that workers are made aware of the positive use of body language as a means of either managing aggression or at least not making the situation worse by inadvertently giving off the wrong signals.

Body language operates at a subliminal level and although not necessarily conscious of it we will often react to it. An example of this may be identified within a group when one person yawns and is quickly followed by someone else yawning. Within aggression it is often the aggressor who takes the lead and the person on the receiving end who begins to mirror the body language of aggression. Examples of this include: the aggressor starts tapping and we start tapping; they stand and we stand; or they point and we point, etc.

Body language is influenced by gender, culture and ethnicity. I am white, male, middle-class and English and, although I have spent more time away from my northern roots than there, my formative years have played their part in the formation of my perceptions. We all function in the world carrying similar elements and we react to others often from these fixed perceptions. When we attempt to interpret body language these elements influence interpretation. The consequence is often a limited perception which can preclude a variety of alternative explanations and may lead to inaccurate perception. This in turn can lead to an inappropriate act on our part which may then inflame a situation. It is important that we stop this from happening by acquainting ourselves with as many of the differences in ways of using body language to communicate as possible. I have included some of the more commonly known differences that exist. However, as the number is infinite, it becomes crucial to openly discuss the differences whenever we come into contact in our work with someone who is from a different background. Talking openly about difference will help us to interpret body language appropriately, thereby avoiding inappropriate responses and also increasing awareness of potentially offensive body messages. It will also help to dispel myth, reduce prejudice and create a greater understanding of individuals, cultures and creeds.

Implications

It is important not to signal 'victim' to the aggressor as this will increase the feeling of power within her/him. It is equally important not to indicate that we are also aggressive as this will be reacted to more often than not with a greater level of aggression. Additionally, there is nothing more infuriating than the person on the receiving end of aggression becoming super-calm or super-cool and giving off signals that indicate a lack of concern or involvement. The aggressor will perceive this as a challenge and will often become more aggressive to elicit a response.

Keeping these points in mind, therefore, the following is a list of fourteen of the more common forms of body language which may be used in the majority of situations to positively influence aggressive behaviour.

1   non-confrontational stances
2   positive use of space
3   touching
4   appearance
5   head movements
6   facial expression
7   eye contact
8   posturing
9   use of hand signals
10   hand to head movements
11   body holding or touching
12   reflective body language
13   repetitive movements
14   potential sexual signals

(At the end of this section I have included an exercise that will allow you to identify all these elements and give you the opportunity of considering your body language within aggression.)

1 Non-confrontational stances

Face-to-face stances will mostly be reacted to as confrontational. Try to stand at a slight angle to the aggressor, without turning away. A simple way to achieve this is to position the feet with one foot slightly in front of the other, ensuring that the weight is on the back foot without actually leaning. The distance between the feet should be approximately 10 centimetres from the front heel to the middle of the back foot. Keep the distance between the feet to this length as open stances often indicate the potential for action to follow. Feet together can be perceived as 'victim' signals.

Try it out until you can feel comfortable with the stance. With the feet positioned in such a manner you will notice that the upper torso is now turned at a slight angle, bringing you away from the confrontational stance.

The rationale is: an aggressive body message often has the aggressor leaning forward, usually with the weight on the front foot. A signal of non-aggression, therefore, is the reverse, but controlled in such a manner that the image portrayed is not one of victim.

Be careful not to move into a T-positional stance whereby the back foot is at a 90-degree angle to the front foot, as this can indicate intransigence and a refusal to be prepared to negotiate.

When sitting, try to ensure that the seats are positioned at an angle of about 45 degrees. Alternatively, if the seats are permanently fixed in a directly opposed position, you can turn slightly to sit at an angle in the seat which can help indicate a non-confrontational stance.

2 Positive use of space

The majority of individuals carry with them an imaginary area which is their defendable space. Should this area be encroached upon, the person may feel invaded, which can create an instinctive adverse reaction. Defendable space changes with situations and feelings of insecurity. Imagine if you were walking down a road during the day and people were passing by on the same side of the road, coming within a few metres of you. You would probably feel unconcerned. Imagine, however, you are in the same road, late at night. The lighting is poor and the road is deserted save for you. You hear a sound some 10 metres behind you. Now, how would you feel? Probably aware, if not anxious. Next let us suggest that you turn and see the vague shape of a person walking purposefully towards you. At this stage, irrespective of the distance involved, you would probably feel threatened.

Space is also influenced by:

• Gender – generally women get closer to other women, men maintain a greater distance from other men, men often like to get closer to women, while women often like to keep men further away.
• Ethnicity – for some people from different ethnic backgrounds close physical proximity is a positive message of a desire to communicate.
• Culture – the establishment within which you work may have established a culture whereby colleagues and service users use close proximity to indicate friendliness.

In my opinion **the average space requirement between you and an aggressor is generally about two arm lengths if standing, and perhaps one-and-a-half arm lengths (at shoulder level) if sitting.** Maintaining this distance between yourself and a person who is becoming aggressive can help to reduce the tension while also providing a safer distance should a punch be thrown.

ACTIVITY 5.1

In order to identify your defendable space, working with a colleague:

At opposite ends of a room stand facing your colleague. Ask your colleague to remain stationary while you walk towards him/her and to give a sign once he/she 'feels' your presence.

Repeat the process with your colleague this time walking towards you.

3 Touching

Another general rule that I advocate concerns the use of touch: **try not to touch the aggressor first as it is usually instantly reacted to with hostility.**

The rationale is: as the invasion of defendable space is often reacted to negatively, the idea of touching another person must indicate a greater escalation of the situation.

In discussions held with many professionals over the sixteen years that I have been training, it has been explained to me that there can be a therapeutic value in touching a person who is exhibiting aggressive behaviour, and that such intervention can enable the person's behaviour to de-escalate. This has usually taken place within units where the use of touch has been discussed and agreed beforehand as a means of calming the individual. When used within these units, touch has been identified as a constructive and caring element and not as a coercive measure to ensure compliance. The guidelines around its use have also been within the framework of 'good practice' identified in the document, *Guidance on Permissible Forms of Control in Children's Residential Care*[1] and the Sir Herbert Laming letter, 'The control of children in the public care: interpretation of the Children Act 1989'.[2]

In situations where the person is not known or where the use of touch has not previously been identified and agreed upon as a calming device, the general rule applies.

Be aware that some low-order touching often takes place by the aggressor as a means of allowing them to more easily physically or verbally assault the person. The aggressor may, for example, innocently brush against, or purposefully barge into, the person. Alternatively, they may prod a shoulder. In situations where the aggressor cannot actually make contact – for example, the worker may operate behind a perspex screen – prodding the screen separating them from their would-be victim is an indication of the same low-order touching.

This low-order touching can often be a signal for higher levels of aggression to follow, either immediately or for an average of up to ninety minutes afterwards – the reason being that for many people it takes a long time to get into the state of aggression, and equally it takes a long time for them to come away from the associated feelings of irritability, frustration and anger. With some people it can be much longer than ninety minutes before these frustrations have passed and they have calmed down. If low-order touching takes place, be on your guard. Within residential or day-care units do not encourage 'play fights', especially between user and carer, which can encourage this freedom of increased aggression.

Be aware that the need to make physical contact by some individuals, as a means of ensuring positive communication, is greater in some cultures than in the traditionally more reserved British culture. Some people, for example, need to hold the wrist and stroke the forearm of the person with whom they are talking. Some may hold shoulders or arms and touch cheeks, while others may shake hands. Within some cultures it is totally unacceptable for a man to make physical contact with a woman who is menstruating, and within some religions it is unacceptable to make physical contact with a person not from the same religion. Incidentally, a number of business schools in Japan are now teaching business personnel how to shake hands, to replace the traditional bow.

ACTIVITY 5.2

Think through, or in a group identify:

1   Under what circumstances does the use of touching become acceptable?

2   What ethnic, gender or cultural differences regarding touch are you aware of?

4 Appearance

What we wear is important. Sometimes our clothes can present an opportunity for an assailant to hurt us. Long dangly earrings through pierced ears may be snatched at and pulled, as may a nose ring; a non-detachable tie, or a necklace without an easy snapping clasp, will give a would-be assailant the opportunity to hold us. Flat shoes are easier to run in. Cotton will rip, allowing us to escape more easily if grabbed. Replace glass lenses with plastic as glass may smash if hit by a fist.

What everyday items do you wear that may be used against you?

It is also important to consider appearance to ensure that:

(a)   We dress appropriately; this does not mean dressing down, which is patronising, but it does mean ensuring that our appearance does not cause offence or provoke negative reaction.
(b)   We do not dress in an ostentatious manner which can reaffirm the difference between the 'haves' and the 'have-nots'.

ACTIVITY 5.3

Identify individually, or in a group discuss:

1   Do you have a dress code in your workplace?

2   What would be the advantages and disadvantages of such a code?

5 Head movements

Have you ever been to a party where you were faced with that person who just prattled on and on and you found yourself repeatedly nodding? Repetitive head nods are reacted to as negative within aggression as they are interpreted as a signal of not listening, or of wanting to be elsewhere. However, **occasional head nods are perceived as active listening** within many cultures, especially when reinforced with appropriate verbal comments or affirmations. Be careful of a side head tilt which can be reacted to as a 'victim' signal. Conversely an almost imperceptible tilt of the head to the side is often used to signal aggression (see also 'Potential sexual signals' p. 84).

A backwards head tilt can be perceived as a superior message and a forwards head tilt as a victim sign.

While ensuring a non-confrontational position, try to **keep your head straight-on to the aggressor**. The only time this rule will not apply may be within those situations where the person is standing above you or sitting lower than you. Here it becomes appropriate to angle your head up or down in order to be straight-on to the aggressor and maintain the impression of remaining in control – looking up without inclining the head increases the amount of eye white shown, giving the impression of a victim; while looking down at the person without inclining the head indicates arrogant superiority.

6 Facial expression

Do not smile in the face of aggression as this will be reacted to as a smirk. Unfortunately this is not as easy as it sounds as the majority of us are conditioned to smile as a way of conveying politeness or friendliness. Alternatively when we feel uncomfortable many of us smile as a means of alleviating discomfort, and when we face aggression we often feel uncomfortable. Aggressive people perceive the world in negative terms and will perceive this smile as a smirk, frequently reacting by demanding '*What are you laughing at?*' or '*What do you find so funny?*'

In order to stop the smile, take a deeper-than-normal intake of breath immediately upon being faced by aggressive behaviour. This will then allow you to come away from the smile while retaining a committed facial expression.

7 Eye contact

Within some cultures it is considered unacceptable to look another person directly in the eye. Some people work on the basis that the eyes are the key to the soul and that it would be impolite to attempt to look into the soul of another. Some people from some ethnic backgrounds will adopt a deferential stance, looking at the floor while communicating with a person in authority. Occasionally the person may almost furtively look up to make fleeting eye contact. Other people may look over the shoulder of the person with whom they are communicating. Within the culture in which I was raised I was brought up to believe that if I asked you a question and you answered me by looking me directly in the eye, then you were honest and straightforward; if you failed to look me in the eye while answering I was taught to believe you were being devious and dishonest. But then I was also brought up to believe that you could always tell the integrity of a man by the shine on his shoes!

Eye contact is usually important in most cultures and with most individuals. However, the type of eye contact will vary. A general rule, therefore, is: try to **establish eye contact without staring**. Staring will often be reacted to as a challenge.

8 Posturing

For many of us, a common reaction when facing aggression is to momentarily FREEZE, and often we have frozen in a stance that may indicate counter-aggression. Without being aware, our upper torso will have risen by one or two centimetres as we have taken in air in readiness for the 'fight or flight' response. At these times the instinctive response is also to tense up and clench the fists. These body messages can be perceived as an aggressive response and will often escalate the situation. Alternatively the freezing process may well be perceived as 'victim' behaviour, which will add power to the aggressor. Use the gentle, deeper-than-normal breathing process previously suggested above (under 'Facial expression'). Slow down your breathing by inhaling and exhaling slightly longer, allowing the torso to relax and allowing you to regain personal control. Breathing more deeply will help to break the freezing process while also slowing the heart rate down, allowing the muscles to relax. It will give you the opportunity to open the hands, lower the shoulders and regain inner control. **Relaxing is one way of signalling non-aggression** as it allows us to stop providing victim or aggressive signals. Be careful, however, not to become too relaxed, as there is nothing more infuriating than providing a nil response to aggression.

9 Use of hand signals

Aggressive acts usually involve a combination of tensing muscles, jabbing fingers or closed fists. The opposite of this, therefore, is to **use gentle, free-flowing, open hand movements**. Do not point at the aggressor, and steer clear of sudden, jerky movements. Wherever possible keep your hands on view and keep your fingers together, as splayed fingers can be interpreted as a sign of anxiety. Hands in pockets can give the impression of disinterest and a thumb stuck in a belt loop or top of a pocket can indicate arrogance or intransigence. When giving a 'stop' sign use one hand only as it is less likely to be misinterpreted – two hands up can indicate the victim signal of 'surrender'. Keep the hand facing the aggressor, fingers together with a slightly cupped palm and, keeping your hand about twenty centimetres from the shoulder (closer than this can often be viewed as anxiety), gently pat the air as you speak. From this position it becomes possible to lower the hand to waist height, and by gently turning the hand palm-up as we continue to communicate verbally we then indicate a desire to negotiate.

10 Hand to head movements

Often when communicating many of us tend to raise a hand towards the mouth, or we may use it to support the chin or even touch our head or hair. **Hand to head movements are often interpreted negatively** in aggression and can be picked up as:

- a sign of anxiety (finger in the mouth)
- loss of patience (hand run through the hair)
- a signal that we are unsure (thumb to one side of the mouth with a finger to the other as we hold the chin)
- a message of disbelief or boredom (hand held in front of the mouth)
- a sexual sign (see p. 84)

Sometimes hand to head movements may lead to nail biting which furthers the perception of anxiety or even fear.

11 Body holding or touching

Often when under verbal attack we fold our arms, and sometimes either hold our arms tightly on the outside, or hold our body on the inside of the arm-fold. It is often instinctive and although it may give comfort **arm or body holding can be reacted to as a victim signal** and is to be avoided if at all possible.

One of the primary reasons for this interpretation concerns the positioning of shoulders and elbows. The aggressor often effectively inflates his/her body posture. In essence the shoulders are raised and the elbows are out – the opposite of this image is depicted in the arm- and body-holding stances where the shoulders are lowered and the elbows are pulled in. A more productive arm-fold is gentle arm-folding with the hands on view.

Another body-holding stance to be avoided is where we hold our arm. We may hold either our forearm – either in front of the body or behind the back – or the upper arm. Once again the elbow and shoulders are pulled in, giving clear 'victim' signals. In order to signal non-aggression, keep the shoulders square (though not square-on to the aggressor – see 'Non-confrontational stances', p. 77) and keep the elbows gently to the side of the body. Holding your own hand and not the forearm will achieve this.

12 Reflective body language

Reflective body language is where the person on the receiving end of aggression adopts the gestures, words and/or mannerisms of the aggressor. It often occurs as an instinctive mirror reflection where the victim unwittingly copies the actions of the aggressor. The technique of reflecting or 'mirroring' body language is frequently used within counselling to signal an understanding of the person being counselled. Indeed some people have used it successfully in aggression as a means of enabling the aggressor to identify with them. The person using the technique would then gradually begin to slow down their reflective body messages, and in many instances the aggressor's own body messages would also begin to abate.

In order to use the technique successfully the person using it must be a skilled practitioner in the use of body language. As the majority of us are not that skilled in the use of body language, my general rule in this area is: **do not use reflective body messages** as they will be perceived as escalatory copycat behaviour and will lead to higher levels of aggression.

13 Repetitive movements

A lot of aggressive behaviour is preceded by some form of repetitive body language. Types of movement such as tapping, prodding, banging or rocking actions are commonplace and they carry their own message of building tension and increasing impatience. Repetitive movement can be accompanied by repetitive language which is often another indication of increasing tension (see p. 47). It may also be accompanied by short, sharp, repetitive breathing, when often the shoulders will move in unison with the breathing.

Repetitive behaviour is often a subconscious method used by many individuals in order to wind themselves up to a point where they can perform the aggressive act. As it is used, albeit subconsciously, as a means of building to aggression, any kind of **repetitive behaviour is likely to be interpreted as a sign of increased tension** and should be avoided. In particular be careful of repetitive foot movements, finger tapping or strumming, pen clicking, pacing and nodding. Keep your movements gentle and free-flowing. Make no jerky or sudden movements, unless of course you are employing one of the defusion methods identified in Part C.

14 Potential sexual signals

Introduction

These ideas and observations are my own and are based upon personal observation and interpretation and discussion with many course participants who have experienced violence.

It is important to be aware that whatever the interpretation placed upon your body language by the aggressor (would-be or otherwise) it does not provide an excuse for behaviour. Just because we may stand in a certain way or wear a certain item of clothing, that does not give the aggressor a right or a reason to be aggressive.

Body language can be sensual and interpreted as sexual even when it is not meant to be so. I believe, therefore, that **it is important not to increase the potential level of frustration and aggression by unwittingly providing the aggressor with a message that they may interpret as provocative.**

The following ideas are provided to allow you to have a means of de-escalating a situation by avoiding subliminal sexual messages which may heighten tension or increase confusion. These messages are not necessarily gender-related, though perhaps some are more frequently identified with one gender.

- **Hair touching or playing with hair**
  Usually a non-conscious act often performed as a means of comfort. Can be identified as a preening act which may be perceived as 'do you like what you see?'

- **Tongue lip-wetting**
  At times of anxiety the lips can become dry and may need wetting. Try to do this when the aggressor is looking away or by bringing the lips together, which is less provocative than the impression of sensuously moving the tongue along or around the lips.

- **Bent knee**
  Frequently identified in women and often with women who after giving birth to a child have carried the child on the hip. It then becomes custom to stand, even after having stopped carrying the child some years before, with a bent knee and a hip extended out. Both are potential sexual signals, one being a sexual sign (bent knee), the other a sexual zone (hip). Try to stand with knee and hip straight if facing aggression.

- **Pelvic movement**
  Men generally stand with hands behind their backs while rocking the pelvic zone towards the person, which can be perceived as arrogant. Women will more frequently rock the pelvic zone sideways, which can give the impression of anxiety. Keep the zone still in the face of aggression.

- **Fingers pointing towards genital area**
  More frequently found within men who loop the thumbs in the belt, or in the trouser pockets. Do not do it as it will be perceived as arrogance or a macho 'come-on'.

- **Adjusting genital area**
  Often an unconscious act. Some men, however, will use this act purposefully to intimidate or provoke a reaction. While it will not necessarily lead to a heightening of arousal, it is often reacted to with disgust, fear, anxiety or hostility.

Whilst the above signals appear the most common, there are others that should also be avoided. Any of the following can heighten tension by increasing arousal:

- adjusting breast area
- finger or pen sucking
- head tilt, especially combined with eye batting
- touching other person, especially gentle stroking on bare skin
- own body touching or stroking
- physical closeness, with or without contact

In order not to increase the potentiality for aggression, a general rule is: try to **avoid sexual signals**, especially in those situations where ongoing contact with a service user is involved.

The following activity is designed to help participants identify many of the body language signals raised within this section. It will give participants the opportunity to consider their own body messages, and the time to allow for any amendments felt desirable.

ACTIVITY 5.4

This is a group exercise involving up to sixteen participants. You will need a room large enough to allow the group to move freely.
   (Note: This activity requires that all participants can read. If any cannot, choose another activity, such as a video group discussion which may be played

back without sound, allowing individuals to examine their own and other members' body language.)

Prepare a set of A5 cards (one for each of the participants) each having a different message, e.g.

YOU FEEL THREATENED BY YOUR PARTNER

YOU FEEL SUPERIOR TO YOUR PARTNER AND WISH TO CONVEY THIS

YOUR PARTNER FINDS YOU ATTRACTIVE AND YOU WISH TO ENCOURAGE THIS

YOU FEEL ANGRY WITH YOUR PARTNER

YOU ARE CONCERNED FOR YOUR PARTNER

If the group comprises an odd number, have one card marked OBSERVER and provide instructions for the person receiving this card – e.g. 'Please watch for . . .' (whichever elements you wish to highlight).

1   Divide the group into two, requesting the participants to stand in two lines directly opposite each other (allow at least two arms' length distance between the lines).

2   Give instructions:

   (a) No talking allowed throughout.
   (b) Each member is to take a card (offered face down), and to read that card but not to say what is written on it.

3   Once cards have been handed out: if OBSERVER card has been provided ask the observer to take a good vantage point at the back of the room.

4   Further instructions:

   (c) Tell the group that the person referred to as PARTNER is not the person they may live with. For the purposes of this exercise it is the person opposite whom they are now standing, and it does not imply a relationship.
   (d) Ask the group to walk around the room while remaining aware of the movements of their 'partner'.
   (e) Upon hearing the word 'Now' individuals are to approach their 'partner' and then freeze in the position best indicated by what is written on their card.

5   Ask individuals to examine their own body position and to remember this, before then requesting the group to come out of their frozen positions and relax.

6   Where used, receive information from OBSERVER.

7   In turn, request each pair to adopt their positions and hold these while the group then interprets the messages being conveyed.

8   Following interpretation by group, request pair to state the messages they were trying to convey.

9 Continue until all pairs have been considered. Help participants to identify the messages covered in Part A.

10 Discuss the ethnic, gender and/or cultural differences that may exist, and of which participants have direct experience (avoid generalised statements that may be pejorative).

KEY POINTS: PART A

1 Body language is an important component within aggression.

2 Staff can make use of positive body language to help convey elements of control in a non-aggressive manner.

3 Body language is influenced by situation, gender, culture and ethnicity.

4 It is important to discuss ethnic, culture and gender differences to diminish ignorance and reduce prejudice.

5 General rules governing body language within aggression are:

☐ Keep movements gentle and free-flowing.

☐ Use open hand communication.

☐ One-hand communication is less likely to be misinterpreted.

☐ Do not smile.

☐ Do not point.

☐ Keep appropriate distance.

☐ Use occasional head nods.

☐ Do not touch the aggressor first.

☐ Establish eye contact without staring.

☐ Breathe deeply and gently.

REFERENCES

1 *Guidance on Permissible Forms of Control in Children's Residential Care*, issued by the Department of Health in April 1993, is a document covering the law relating to interventions to restrain or restrict the liberty of children in care. It offers guidance for workers in such areas as the use of physical presence, holding and touching.

2 The Laming letter, dated February 1997, entitled 'The control of children in the public care: interpretation of the Children Act 1989', was circulated by the Social Services Inspectorate to all social services departments to further clarify the guidance issued, with particular reference to the professional role, powers and objectives of staff.

KEY READING

Cohen, D. (1992) *Body Language in Relationships*. Sheldon Press.

Morris, D. (1994) *Bodytalk: A World Guide to Gestures*. Cape.

Quilliam, S. (1994) *Child Watching: A Parents' Guide to Children's Body Language*. Ward Lock.

Wilson, G. (1996) *Winning with Body Language*. Bloomsbury.

PART B

ASSERTIVENESS

Have you ever been in those situations where afterwards you walked away knowing you had let the person get away with something, and wishing you had been able to say or do something to have managed it better? Aggressive behaviour is not restricted to service users; sometimes a fellow professional or a colleague may be hostile, offensive or aggressive; and sometimes it may even be a manager.

On occasion we may fail to address the behaviour with the person simply because it is so unexpected or we fear that by doing so we may make the situation worse for ourselves.

SCENARIO

Judith had spent weeks of her spare time putting together a risk assessment document on the potential danger of violence for her and her colleagues. She did it in her spare time because her manager refused to allow her the time required. Eventually she forwarded the following document to the Head of Service:

Dear Mr Coombes,

I am a residential worker working at Davis Heights Children's and Families Centre. I was asked by the staff at the centre to help identify areas in our work which could provide the potential for violence and which in the opinion of the staff at the centre should be risk-assessed.

In all we are concerned about the following areas.

Staff have received no training on managing violence.

No one is aware of a reporting procedure for identifying levels of violence within the home.

Many serious incidents are not reported, including one where a worker had suffered bruising from having a chair thrown at her.

Supervision is irregular. Staffing levels are low, requiring one worker to be alone with up to ten children.

The staff at Davis Heights would be pleased if these issues could be addressed.

Judith signed the document on behalf of all the staff and forwarded a copy to her direct line manager.

Upon receiving the document her manager was livid. He stormed into the room where she was working with a group of children, slammed the document down and shouted 'How dare you send this without coming to me? It's a load of bloody rubbish. And you're in trouble. Now what have you got to say for yourself?'

Judith usually considered herself to be a strong woman but she was taken completely aback and was unable to respond. When she did respond a few hours later by asking to see her manager, she made the mistake of focusing her discussion upon the contents of her letter and her reasons for sending it to the Head of Service. As a consequence she was told she would have her work scrutinised in the future!

ACTIVITY 5.5

In a group identify:

1 What would you have done if you had been the subject of such behaviour?

2 How could Judith best manage the situation now?

First of all, if anything like the above happens in your work, be aware that you do have the opportunity of using your agency's disciplinary procedures. This is unacceptable behaviour by a manager. (See also Chapter 6 on 'Bullying at work'.) Secondly, should this happen, you can also choose to manage it without caving-in and without responding aggressively or defensively. The method proposed is an assertiveness technique which may be used either immediately (with practice) or within a period of up to three days. If more time has elapsed I suggest you forget about dealing with it assertively, as time changes perception, and what may have achieved immense proportions for you may have been forgotten by the aggressor.

In the above scenario Judith did what many of us would do. She failed to consider the process involved within the act of aggression. Judith concentrated upon the content of the information being given to her by the line manager, and in doing so failed to concentrate upon the key issue – the manner of delivery of the information.

The processes in aggression

1 Task versus behaviour

Whenever we face verbal forms of aggression we are usually facing two distinct processes:

A. What the aggressor is saying
B. How the aggressor is expressing the information

A. What the aggressor is saying

Often the information being given is related to the performance of the worker: '*You promised you'd write that letter*' or '*It's your fault. It wouldn't have happened if you'd have . . .*' Or it could be a personal comment – '*You're worthless*' – or related to someone or something dear to the worker: '*This is a load of rubbish.*'

Irrespective of the information provided, consider that a part of the process is for the aggressor to bring us into the aggression. Be aware that the aggressor will effectively throw out verbal 'hooks' upon which to snag us and then reel us into the aggressive act. At a subliminal level the aggressor does not want their behaviour managed; they want us to argue with them. Once we are caught on any of the verbal 'hooks', we become a part of the process and not a manager of it. It is the task of the aggressor to effectively snag us. Let us therefore identify the content or information given by the aggressor as the TASK (i.e. the task of the aggressor to make us a part of the process). Do not respond to the TASK issue(s), at least not initially.

B. How the aggressor is expressing the information

The manner of presentation will usually involve shouting, swearing, banging or some other aggressive act. Alternatively, it could be presented in a cold and calculating manner where the tone of voice carries its own information, ranging from threat to superior hostility and even sarcasm. This is the BEHAVIOUR of the aggressor and it is this element that should be addressed first. If we ignore behaviour it will frequently get worse. Unfortunately, all too often it is this element that is ignored.

Example of BEHAVIOUR being ignored and TASK issue being dealt with

Service user shouting over the telephone: '*What the hell are you lot doing? My mother hasn't eaten for days and all you can do is talk!*'
Care manager: '*We're trying our best, Mr Jones.*'
Service user still shouting: '*Well your best isn't good enough.*' The behaviour of the service user now escalates into a threat: '*If you don't get something sorted today, there's going to be trouble!*'

ACTIVITY 5.6

Individually or in a group, identify:

1 What is the care manager doing wrong in this scenario?

2 What should the care manager do next to best manage the situation?

3 How would you deal with the above situation?

4 What would be the potential outcome of the method you have employed to manage the situation?

A PROCESS IN AGGRESSION

TASK	AND	BEHAVIOUR
A (Content or hooks to catch worker) 'What the hell are you lot doing? My mother hasn't eaten for days and all you can do is talk!'	= 1	(Manner of presentation of information)
	=	Shouting
B Response: We're trying our best, Mr Jones' (worker is hooked)	= 2	Behaviour is ignored
C 'If you don't get something sorted today, there's going to be trouble!'	= 3	Behaviour worsens into threat

The primary focus of the worker when faced with aggression is to deal with the BEHAVIOUR and leave the TASK until later, even when the task issue is work-related.

Example of work-related TASK issue being left and the BEHAVIOUR being dealt with

Service user shouting: '*What the hell are you lot doing? My mother hasn't eaten for days and all you can do is talk!*'
Care manager: '*Mr Jones, stop shouting at me and tell me about your mother's situation.*'

What is the possible outcome from this interaction?

Not getting caught on the task but dealing with BEHAVIOUR is crucial. The manner in which we deal with the behaviour is of equal importance, as we can remain in charge of, and not become a part of, the other processes involved.

2 Forms of behaviour

There are three ways in which aggression can be responded to. We can all be:

(a) **Aggressive.** Unfortunately we often meet aggression with aggression and, although it is a way of communicating, the chance of it effectively managing aggressive behaviour within another is perhaps dependent upon circumstance, size and ability. In the majority of situations I strongly advise against the use of aggression as a means of managing aggression. It is not constructive communication and it can store up problems for the future.

(b) **Passive.** It is often infuriating to deal with a person who is not prepared to speak up for themselves or the situation facing them, or who will not make a decision or take a stand over an issue. Passivity can frequently lead to feelings of anger and expressions of aggression – if we let people walk over us they will continue to do so.

(c) **Assertive.** A commonly held belief is that assertive and aggressive behaviours are very similar. Additional mythology suggests that assertiveness is only required by those people who are passive. In fact, assertiveness is a different method of communicating. It is the middle road which effectively fuses aggressive and passive responses into a unique style. It is the approach that is more likely to effectively and constructively manage aggression.

Aggressive and passive reactions are instinctive responses within aggression, and they are the frequent reactions given by the majority of individuals experiencing aggression. They are in effect the 'fight or flight' responses identified by anthropologists. Such reactions are unlikely to be effective in managing aggression.

Assertiveness is often a learned approach and frequently requires individuals to rethink the manner in which they communicate, maybe even changing the order of words, the tone used and emphasis employed. It also requires on occasion a change in the body language used by the worker when facing aggression. (See Part A.)

3 The assertive components when facing aggression

Assertiveness is used in a variety of situations, and when attempting to manage aggressive behaviour there are ten elements that need to be taken into account:

(i)   **An ability to manage personal anxiety**
      Managing personal anxiety is a fundamental starting point, because if we cannot manage our own anxiety it will be difficult to manage any situation.

- Beforehand – talk it over with someone and work out what you are going to say and how you are going to say it. Practise saying the actual words you intend to use, if you can.
- During – take a breath before you say or do anything. Often at these times we are anxiety-driven and we blurt out the first thing on our minds. The breath will give us the time to think of the appropriate words.
- After – acknowledge that you can feel fragile or vulnerable, and take time out for yourself to make sure you are all right. Take a break, even if only for a few minutes. Talk it over with someone. It is no use going from one difficult situation straight into another because you will carry over some emotion which might then come out on the next person.

It is also important to manage the anxiety often created when experiencing aggression from a 'person in power', or in those situations where we fear that by addressing the behaviour we will either make the situation worse or create an irreparable gulf between us and the other person.

(ii) **The use of 'I' language**
      Using 'I' allows the aggressor to perceive an individual, and it is harder to damage an individual than the anonymous 'we', 'us' or 'our'. Use the aggressor's name if you know it. Give your name if you feel able. The use of 'I' also helps the aggressor to obtain a sense of responsibility for the consequences of their behaviour.

(iii) **Clarity**
      Know what you want to happen and say it. Deal with the BEHAVIOUR; leave the TASK till later. Avoid ambiguity. Know the feeling the behaviour is generating within yourself and be prepared to articulate this.

(iv) **The ability to be specific**
      Use the words that best describe the behaviour or situation before you. We are often taught that it is impolite to be specific and we often generalise as a means of being polite. So instead of saying '*Put the gun down so I can speak to you*', we might say something like '*Come on, this isn't going to achieve much.*' Using the words to describe the behaviour gives the aggressor greater opportunity to change that behaviour.

(v)   **The use of direct communication**
      Sometimes we make the assumption that the aggressor knows what they are doing

– that they know they are having an impact upon us – and we fail to address the behaviour. Stop making such assumptions. Instead make statements about the behaviour, as a way of giving the person the opportunity to stop or change the behaviour. Stop pussyfooting around and make the statement(s) as soon as possible.

(vi) **The art of gentle precision**

Be precise and polite. Use short sentences and keep the sentences gentle. A good way of achieving this is to consider the appropriate use of the word *'Please'*, but be careful. *'Please'* used at the beginning or the end of a sentence can be perceived as 'victim'. Try putting it in the middle, where it will be perceived as polite, which is often disarming in the face of aggression. Repeat if necessary, but do not become over-repetitive.

Assertiveness training often suggests using the 'broken record' approach whereby we continue to repeat the message. When facing aggression, however, do not over-repeat, as this may escalate the situation.

(vii) **An inner confidence**

So many times when we face aggression the mental impression we give ourselves is negative. This will not help as the feeling can be picked up by the aggressor. Say to yourself *'I can manage this'*, without becoming blasé. This inner confidence will then be conveyed in a positive approach.

(viii) **A positive approach**

Take a positive approach in what you do and say. Take a deeper-than-normal intake of breath, or if frozen in a posturing stance, gently exhale. Slow down your breathing. This will influence the heart rate and allow your movements to be gentle and free-flowing. It will also release the tension in the throat muscles, allowing the saliva to flow, and enable you to speak without a quiver in the voice.

(ix) **An awareness of own feelings**

The behaviour facing us will, for the majority, have an impact upon us. It is important to be aware of this because it often becomes necessary to control our own feelings before we can expect to control those of another person. Internal identification and acknowledgement of our feeling(s) allow us this control. Awareness also gives us the opportunity of using the feelings appropriately (see 'An assertiveness technique for managing aggression', p. 94).

(x) **Not asking questions**

A part of the process of many acts of aggression is to ask questions: *'What are you looking at? . . . What do you find so funny? . . . Are you looking for a fight?'*

Asking questions can in effect become a psychological trigger, triggering the other person into believing that you too are being aggressive. Conversely, asking questions can create the victim image – *'Would you mind not doing that?'* – as well as giving the aggressor the opportunity to expand their aggressive behaviour. Making a statement about the behaviour and requesting the aggressor to stop the behaviour provides information and offers a boundary. Do not ask questions until the behaviour is dealt with.

The next time you witness aggression, listen to the process of questions being asked.

---

4 An assertiveness technique for managing aggression

Keeping the above elements in mind, one assertive technique for managing some aggressive behaviours involves four stages. Each stage is linked and follows relatively swiftly. The idea with this approach is not to give the aggressor the opportunity to argue further or to continue with their behaviour. It is based upon the fact that the aggressor has the advantage of surprise, and the person on the receiving end is usually shocked and overwhelmed. Secondly, the balance of power in the situation is usually with the aggressor. This technique redresses that imbalance and allows the opportunity of a WIN/WIN outcome for both people. It does require practice and will not work in every situation:

(a) make a statement about the BEHAVIOUR
(b) state the IMPACT of the behaviour upon you
(c) request aggressor to STOP the behaviour
(d) return to the TASK or change the subject

(a) Make a statement about the BEHAVIOUR

Frequently we ask questions. At this initial point, avoid doing so. Be clear, precise, direct, specific, etc., and use the person's name if you know it: '*David, you're swearing.*' Keep your tone gentle, your voice relatively low and yet firm.

(b) State the IMPACT of the behaviour upon you

This is something that many people find difficult to do as it often implies giving away personal information. Also it is often felt that to confirm the impact is to reinforce the power within the aggressor. Think, however, have you ever lost your temper and shouted at someone, only to regret the act an hour or so later, thinking that you may have hurt or upset the other person? Effectively this verbal association between behaviour and impact can eliminate the time gap. Furthermore, if we are to give the person the opportunity to be responsible for the behaviour, it becomes important to allow them to have direct confirmation that their behaviour is creating damage. If we do not say we are being damaged, how can we expect them to know?

The association between behaviour and impact is a technique that will not work in every situation and it becomes a judgement call. It can, however, work in many situations: '*David, your swearing is upsetting me*', or '*David, your swearing is making me feel angry*', or even, '*David, your swearing is offensive.*'

(c) Request aggressor to STOP the behaviour

Imagine you are angry and you are becoming increasingly frustrated by some injustice that you feel is being carried out. Your frustration reaches boiling point and you suddenly stand and shout at the person carrying out the injustice. The person responds to this by saying '*Keep calm*'. I imagine your reaction might be to become (at least initially) more demonstrative and you may well reply '*I am bloody calm!*'

Using the word 'stop' provides a clear boundary. Say gently: 'Stop.' Using 'please' at this stage can also be productive (see 'The art of gentle precision', p. 93).

The technique now appears as:

'David your (<u>behaviour</u>) is (<u>impact</u>) (<u>request to stop</u>) . . .'

'David your <u>swearing</u> is <u>intimidating</u> me, please <u>stop</u> . . .'

(d) Return to the TASK or change the subject

Next, before the aggressor has time to think and/or argue, add the last stage. If the aggressor was referring to a situation, an event or piece of work, refer back to the element raised. If this is not possible, change the subject.

'David, your swearing is intimidating me, please stop. Now tell me about your . . . (<u>situation being shouted about</u>) . . .'

This element of the technique allows the person the opportunity to save face. They may choose to apologise for their behaviour or they may choose to ignore the apology and concentrate upon the issue. Either way the person now knows where they stand.

Example of technique

Service user shouting: '*What the hell are you lot doing? My mother hasn't eaten for days and all you can do is talk!*'
Care manager: '*Mr Jones, you're shouting. I find it offensive. Please, stop shouting and tell me about your mother's situation.*'

Let us now reconsider the previous scenario involving Judith and her manager (see p. 88):

. . . Upon receiving the document her manager was livid. He stormed into the room where she was working with a group of children, slammed the document down and shouted 'How dare you send this without coming to me? It's a load of bloody rubbish. And you're in trouble. Now what have you got to say for yourself?'

ACTIVITY 5.7

Individually or in a group:

1 Identify the words and manner of delivery Judith could use to address this situation, using the above assertiveness technique.

2 Next consider the following vignettes and decide how the situations may be managed assertively.

Vignette 1

You are working in a residential care home for older people, escorting an older woman, Mary, who is using a zimmer frame to see her daughter. Her daughter has just walked into the building and is waiting by the door. Another resident who has been agitated all morning rushes past, barging into Mary, knocking her to the floor. The daughter storms forward almost screaming: 'Look what you've done. You stupid cow.'

Vignette 2

You are in a chair reading a departmental memo. A senior manager in your agency who has a reputation for touching people has walked up behind you. (S)he leans over you, in an effort to see the document, and fondles your shoulders.

Vignette 3

You are new in your position. A colleague who has been at the unit for a number of years has been making snide comments about you for a few days now. Today (s)he does it again.

Vignette 4

You are having a telephone conversation with a psychiatrist who expects you to reverse a decision made at a case conference. The psychiatrist is becoming increasingly annoyed and coldly states: 'Well, if you don't visit and she dies it'll be your fault.'

There may be situations where it becomes inappropriate to use a verbal assertive approach:

Vignette 5

You are alone on a train sitting by the window. The rest of the carriage is deserted. A man you do not know chooses to sit next to you, touching you with his leg and leaning towards you.

In the above vignette it becomes inappropriate to attempt to use a verbal method to manage the behaviour because to do so is to invite the aggressor to become involved. In such situations stand and walk purposefully away.

5 An assertiveness technique for handling negative criticism

Criticism is often difficult for many of us to handle, as it often takes us back to a period in our childhood when, instead of aspects of behaviour being criticised, the attack was on the image of ourselves: *'You're naughty'* or *'You're a bad boy . . . You're hopeless . . . You're no good . . .'*, etc. In fact what was usually being criticised was an aspect of ourselves: a behaviour. As children it is difficult to manage this attack on 'self', simply because we do not have the communication skills to do so. Also when children attempt to address it they usually become the subject of more criticism, or are shunned or punished in some way. The message provided is that it is therefore somehow wrong to attempt to manage it, or that by attempting to manage it, it only gets worse. This impression is frequently carried into adulthood, so when we are criticised we usually react to it as we did as children and either fail to address it or address it in an inappropriate manner.

1   Listen to what is being said. This is important because often we may reject it, become angry or defensive. 'You're always late.'

2   Ask yourself: 'Is there any truth in it?'

3   If YES ↓

    (a) Acknowledge it and use the word being used to criticise: 'Yes it's true I was <u>late</u>'

    (b) Redefine it into a smaller aspect: 'Yes, it's true I was late <u>today and I may have been late yesterday</u>'

    (c) Give a positive proposal: <u>'But I won't be late tomorrow'</u>

    (d) Take action

If NO ↓

    (a) Reject it using the word 'No': '<u>No</u>, that's not true, I was not late'

    (b) Give evidence: <u>'I was at that meeting you asked me to attend'</u>

    (c) Put it back to the person, seeking clarification: <u>'But you seem to have the impression that I am always late – can you tell me where that comes from?'</u>

Incidentally, adults who care for children are now being taught to criticise behaviour – e.g. 'What you just did was naughty', and not 'You're naughty'. It is hoped that future generations will find it easier to manage criticism.

KEY POINTS: PART B

Assertiveness:

- ☐   Is for the majority a learned response.
- ☐   Involves both verbal and non-verbal skills.
- ☐   Is a specific method of communicating.
- ☐   May take a rethinking of the manner in which we presently communicate.
- ☐   Will not be appropriate in some situations.
- ☐   Requires management of our own reaction.
- ☐   Is not easy.
- ☐   Requires practice.

By now you should be aware of the different forms of behaviour available to anyone to help manage aggression. You know of the component parts that make up assertiveness and you have a technique for managing some of the covert as well as the more overt forms of aggression. You also have a technique for managing criticism.

KEY READING

Bishop, S. (1996) *Develop Your Assertiveness*. Kogan Page.
Lemon, C. (1997) *Assert Yourself*. Gower.
Lindenfield, G. (rev. edn, 2000) *Confident Children: Help Children Feel Good about Themselves*.
   Thorsons.

PART C

DEFUSION TECHNIQUES

Introduction

Defusion techniques are verbal and non-verbal methods of communication designed to manage aggressive behaviour while ensuring personal safety. They will not work in every situation and different approaches will be required for different people. They deal with the immediate situation by taking the heat out of it and are therefore both an important component within a worker's communication skills and a significant element in managing aggression. For the best results practise using them, perhaps in role-plays, with work colleagues or by yourself, to familiarise yourself with them so that you are comfortable with a variety of different approaches. You will probably need to use a number of the techniques within any one situation, always remembering, however, that **sometimes nothing works** because some people have behaviours that are unmanageable.

   For the majority of occasions there are things that you can say and/or do that will help to manage the aggressive behaviour and/or the situation.

Defusion techniques:

1   MAINTAINING SELF-CONTROL
2   USE OF POSITIVE BODY LANGUAGE
3   SITTING DOWN
4   POSITIVE WORDS AND PHRASES
5   BOUNDARY WORDS/INFORMATION
6   ACKNOWLEDGEMENT
7   DIVERSION
8   IDENTIFYING PAST STRENGTHS
9   GAINS and LOSSES
10   CONCERN
11   HUMOUR
12   NON-RESPONSE
13   LEAVING
14   DISTRACTION

1 Maintaining self-control

Maintaining personal control is crucial when faced with aggression, though it is not an easy thing to do. The aggressor may be breathing rapidly and shallowly, their movements uneven and jerky, their tone hard and their sentences clipped. You, at this stage, can instinctively either become frozen with fear, or react with aggression. To change this instinctive reaction, take one deeper-than-normal intake of breath and gently exhale. This action will allow you to feel more in control and will also give you enough time to think through what you are going to say or do next.

Some people who have been held hostage have explained afterwards that in order to maintain personal control they played an imaginary record over in their mind which helped them to respond appropriately.

The record was something like:

'*I can get through this. Slow down my breathing. Look for my exits. Relax my muscles. Think what am I going to say next. Breathe deeply.*'

If we can remain in control of our own emotions we convey the message that we can help the aggressor to control their emotions. If on the other hand we are drawn into the process and react from fear or anger, or even if we become under- or non-responsive, this will generally escalate the situation.

2 Use of positive body language

Maintaining personal control is an internal process that can help provide the confidence to manage the situation. The use of positive body language is the outward expression of this inner confidence (see Part A).

3 Sitting down

In many situations it becomes possible to judge the moment when the aggression is at the point of escalation – that moment when the behaviour is moving from truculence into a more strident form. At this point (if not before) sit down and invite the aggressor to sit down with an open hand gesture. Only sit down if you feel confident. It is a demonstrative model which allows the aggressor to perceive de-escalation. The act is a clear signal of non-aggression and a sign of negotiation.

Many people feel that sitting may be identified by the aggressor as a 'victim' signal. However, ask yourself, how many times do you see people fighting when they are standing and how many times do you see a person fighting who is seated?

There are occasions when the person who is aggressive is already seated, as in the case of a wheelchair user, for example. In such instances, try sitting at the same height or even in a slightly lower seat than the person, without patronising the individual concerned. Sit at an angle in a non-confrontational manner (see Part A, p. 77).

Do not sit down if physical assault is imminent or if you feel insecure.

4 Positive words and phrases

While some words and phrases can have the effect of making a situation worse, others can be more productive in decreasing the level of aggression being expressed.

Words and phrases to avoid	*Alternatives to try*
Don't be silly/stupid . . .	<u>You are important and what you do is important</u>
It's not as bad as all that . . .	<u>It sounds really awful</u>
You're not going to achieve much like that . . .	<u>Stop [behaviour] and tell me what you want</u>
Can't . . . Mustn't . . . Shouldn't . . .	<u>Can . . . Could . . . Would . . .</u>

Negative words only add to the negative state of aggression being expressed. Replace with positive ones. For example, the expression, 'I can't help you if you are shouting at me', can work for you, but the expression is not as powerful as the positive '<u>I can help you if you stop shouting</u>'.

Understand or Know	<u>See</u> or <u>Hear</u>

A popular word used within social care is 'understand'. However, when facing aggression do not use it because it often leads to the negative response, 'No you don't'.

You lot . . .	<u>Name of individuals (if known)</u>
People like *you* . . .	<u>Name of person (if known)</u>
We/our/us	

It is easier to damage an anonymous entity rather than an individual, and aggressively behaved people use words to enable them to perceive anonymity (see p. 47). Anonymous and generalised plurals such as 'we' aid in that process, as do accusatory or dismissive words such as 'you' or 'you lot'. Replace with:

	'I' and <u>names</u> wherever possible, e.g. <u>I'm Ray and I'm here on behalf of . . .</u>
Yes, but . . .	<u>Yes</u>
Forms of jargon, e.g.:	Simple explanation/language
I hear what you're saying . . .	<u>It sounds awful</u>
I can see where you're coming from . . .	<u>Yes, I see</u>
With respect . . .	[avoid any patronising]

ACTIVITY 5.8

Brainstorm:

What jargon is common usage in your work?

What does the use of jargon mean?

---

5 Boundary words/information

Many of us like to know where our boundaries are, including what we can and cannot do, and a clear boundary word is 'No'. The value of the word 'No' cannot be understated. As children it helped us to identify boundaries, and with some lower levels of aggression its use can be extremely valuable. In some instances, however, the word 'No' can be perceived as a barrier rather than a boundary and can be reacted to with increased hostility. Try therefore using alternative ways of giving the same information. For example:

Service user:	'I'm going out.'
Care worker:	'No you're not.'
Alternative answer:	<u>'I know you want to and it is difficult staying in . . .'</u>

ACTIVITY 5.9

In a group:

Identify those occasions where the use of the word 'No' has sparked an even greater level of aggression.

Now identify an alternative way of conveying the same information but without using 'No'.

Note that using the word 'No' when facing aggression can often be very therapeutic for the victim, especially following a serious incident, and therefore I advocate its use when faced with extreme forms of violence. However, for less extreme forms of aggression it is often advisable to use alternatives.

As well as being a clear boundary word in its own right, the word 'Stop' is an alternative to 'No'. 'Stop' will often be perceived more positively and is less likely to inflame a situation, especially when used in linking a description of behaviour to a positive outcome for changing that behaviour (see 'Gains and Losses', p. 105).

Some organisations working with people with special needs, where the use of language is not available, use colour-coded cards which convey the same 'boundary' information. A red card may indicate the requirement to stop the behaviour, while a green card may indicate encouragement to continue.

6 Acknowledgement

In many instances the aggressor is providing a message not only in the content of what they are saying but also in the manner in which they are expressing themselves. If the way a person is expressing themselves is ignored the behaviour is likely to get worse. However, by making an acknowledgement of one or more of the elements involved in the manner of expression, you are saying to the aggressor that the message has been received and they need not therefore continue to express themselves in that way.

Acknowledge one or more of three elements:

THE BEHAVIOUR	'David, stop *banging the table* and . . .'
THE SITUATION	'David, your mother died, it's understandable that you're acting like this . . .'
THE EMOTION	'You sound really angry . . .'

Whilst acknowledging either the BEHAVIOUR or the SITUATION can be valuable, because (a) some people are unaware of their actions and will actually apologise once they recognise what they are doing, and (b) some people are unable to vocalise their own situation, perhaps the most powerful element of the three to vocalise is the EMOTION, anger.

Acknowledgement of anger can create a number of reactions within the aggressor which may then be worked with.

First, the use of the word ANGER may provoke a cathartic release, encouraging the aggressor to erupt, effectively ridding the person of their built-up tension. Secondly, using the word ANGER actually values the emotion experienced by not denying the right to be angry. Thirdly, it can allow the aggressor to become aware of a previously unidentified emotion. And finally it demonstrates that you are not afraid of the emotion. For example:

> Angry service user stomping around and shouting about the service.
>
> Worker intercedes: 'David, I can see you're angry.'
>
> Service user responds with a louder outburst: 'Too bloody right I am!'

At this point it is necessary for the worker to regain the advantage by a further acknowledgement of both the situation and the behaviour:

> Worker: 'Yes, I can see that. But you don't have to shout. Come on, sit down and let's get it sorted.'

If you are concerned that using the word ANGER too boldly may provoke an extreme reaction from the aggressor, making you feel even more vulnerable, put the word in more obliquely. For example:

> 'David, I can see things aren't working out for you, but getting angry isn't going to help. Come on, sit down and let's talk about it.'

7 Diversion

Diversion is the constructive use of the element of change, and there are three options available to anyone who employs this technique:

(a)   Changing the topic
(b)   Changing the subject of the aggression
(c)   Changing the environment within which the aggression is occurring

(a) Changing the topic

Anyone who has a young child will know how this form of diversion works:

> Child demanding: 'I want this. I want this. I want this.'
>
> Carer: 'What's on telly tonight?'

The simplicity of the technique is that it can immediately change the situation by creating confusion within the other person. Imagine the confusion created within the aggressor in the following example:

> Adolescent boy shouting: 'I want my money! I want it now!'
>
> Care worker responds: 'How did the Arsenal do last night?'

Changing the subject can create confusion, but once the confusion has been created and the aggression has momentarily abated, it becomes necessary to immediately move on, otherwise the aggression is more likely to be accelerated:

Adolescent boy shouting: 'I want my money! I want it now!'

Care worker responds: 'How did the Arsenal do last night?'

Adolescent boy no longer shouting incredulously responds: 'What?'

Care worker: 'Now that you've stopped shouting, let's sit down and talk about your money.'

Only use this technique once in any one encounter, otherwise it will be spotted for what it is – a manipulative tool to stop the behaviour. Try also to use it sparingly, especially within residential or day-care settings where it may have less of an impact upon other service users who may have witnessed its usage.

(b) Changing the subject of the aggression

Sometimes it is you who the service user is aggressive towards, whereas they may not be aggressive towards another member of staff. This may be due to one of a thousand reasons, such as a personality clash, or you may remind the aggressor of someone else, etc. It is important to consider that you may not be the appropriate person to manage this behaviour and that sometimes it is appropriate to involve someone else.

In situations where you are being shouted at and you have a colleague with you, try turning to that colleague and saying: *'This is difficult, can you take over?'* Make sure that you have discussed this tactic with your colleague beforehand, otherwise they may feel they have been dumped unfairly with a difficult situation.

Alternatively, if the aggressive service user has a relative or friend with them, it can sometimes help to invite that person to become involved: *'This is difficult. Mrs Jones, can you do something?'* By taking this action you are giving the friend or relative the opportunity of helping and not giving them the easy options of either simply witnessing the situation or being drawn into it and becoming an additional aggressor.

(c) Changing the environment

Sometimes environment can encourage aggression (see 'Ecological theories', p. 23) and a few minor changes may make the environment less threatening.

Besides the physical environment, other people within the same environment can:

* create a situation where the aggressor cannot stop their behaviour because to do so would be to lose face
* provide an audience to which the aggressor will play
* give encouragement to continue

If there are other people around, try to remove the aggressor (without physical contact) from the audience, always ensuring that you are not placing yourself at greater risk. If it is not possible to move the aggressor, ask a colleague to become involved with the audience, redirecting their attention from the aggressor while you deal with his/her behaviour. The act of bringing in a colleague will also change the environment.

8 Identifying past strengths

Many people who are in a hostile state are in a state of negativity, and by giving the person the reminder of when they were in a positive state we can allow them to refocus upon this. This is a technique that also rewards positive rather than criticising negative behaviour. If we have some knowledge of the person, referring to this knowledge can often help. Consider the following example:

> Sean, a young man with learning difficulties, was beginning to become frustrated while attempting to draw. Suddenly his behaviour became extreme as he scribbled furiously on his pad. The care worker involved picked up a picture from last week's pile and gently said, 'Hey Sean, hang on. Look here's one you did last week. Let's see how you did that.' Sean stopped his action and was able to refocus upon the previous achievement.

Sometimes it may be as simple as referring to a previous encounter:

> Service user demanding action begins to shout.
>
> Care worker responds by saying: 'Hang on Mr Teek. I saw you last week and you didn't have to shout then. And we got it sorted. And you don't have to shout now.'
>
> Mr Teek stops his behaviour, remembering the previous positive encounter.

Or even a positive past memory:

> Without realising the room was now occupied, Jean, a care officer in a home for older people, walked into the bedroom and was confronted by a man in his eighties who raised his walking stick. 'What the hell are you doing?' he shouted. Jean had been told that the room was to be occupied by a Mr Simons, a man with senile dementia whose day-to-day memory was poor, but whose long-term memory was amazingly acute. Looking around the room she noticed the framed picture of a cat on the dressing table. 'Is that your pet cat?' she asked, walking over to the picture.
> 'Oh, yes, that's my Timmy', replied Mr Simons, lowering the stick and walking over to the picture himself.

9 Gains and losses

Most of us have had our behaviour threatened with potential negative outcomes at different stages from our early childhood. For example, how many of us have heard our parents say *'if you don't stop that I'll belt you'*, or *'carry on and you're in for a good smacking'*? We are mostly therefore accustomed to the concept of being reminded of what we may lose if we do not stop.

We are not as accustomed to the concept of being told what we stand to gain should we change our bad behaviour into good.

Reminding us of our gains prior to our losses within the situation is valuable because:

(a)   it is unexpected and therefore disarming
(b)   it rewards good behaviour
(c)   it gives the aggressor responsibility for the outcome

A simple example is: '*Stop shouting and I'll see what I can do.*'
   This technique has been successfully employed over the telephone. For example: '*Stop shouting and I'll stay listening but if you don't stop shouting I'm going to hang up.*'
   If using the potential threat, '*If you don't stop I'll . . .*', you must be prepared to carry out your proposed action, so do not make threats that you are not prepared to see through.
   Where possible give service users who you know are likely to lose their temper the opportunity of receiving a reward for maintaining good behaviour prior to any difficult meetings. For example: '*I know it's going to be difficult for you, David, but if you can get through the whole of that meeting without losing your temper then I will take you swimming.*'

10 Concern

Another disarming technique is the expression of concern, which is unexpected as mostly the aggressor will expect either an aggressive or a passive response. Expressing concern can be achieved in at least three ways:

(a)   First, using the word 'sorry' can be productive. However, it must be meant and must therefore carry the weight of sincerity with it. If it is not your fault do not feel you have to apologise, but you can still use the word effectively: '*David, I'm truly sorry this has happened.*' Alternatively, if it is your fault: '*I'm sorry I kept you waiting.*'
   Do not overuse the word 'sorry'. It is especially overused within a British culture when we apologise every time someone barges into us, or we use it to ask a question. In aggression, therefore, do not use it more than three times in any one encounter, as it will lose impact and be misinterpreted as a manipulative tool to stop behaviour.
(b)   Secondly, an empathetic approach can be effective, whereby we allow the aggressor to identify that we perceive the world through his/her eyes: '*I can see it's difficult for you. I'd be shouting too if this happened to me*', or '*Yes, it really is awful.*' A powerful word to use to demonstrate a show of concern is 'Yes'.
(c)   Thirdly, demonstrating an active listening technique can be most constructive. This may be achieved by repeating to the person the information they are giving you: '*So let me get this right, what you are saying is . . .*'
   Alternatively, use positive affirmations to prove you are listening, such as: '*Yes/this sounds important/right/ermm.*' Combine this with positive body language, such as the use of occasional head nods and establishing eye contact without staring.

Additionally, the taking and giving of information are a demonstrative show of concern.

11 Humour

The use of humour can stop aggressive behaviour, but it is also one of the most dangerous ways because humour is readily open to misinterpretation. Do not use humour at the expense of the aggressor, or their situation, and do not use humour if you are not practised or skilled in its use.

The use of humour can also be perceived as rewarding bad behaviour, and if you are to use it to quell aggression I would strongly advocate, wherever possible, returning to the person afterwards (without placing yourself at risk) to make the person aware that their behaviour was unacceptable.

CASE STUDY

In a day centre for people with learning difficulties lunch had been served and everyone was seating themselves at their tables. The noise level was constant as Kylie sat next to her key worker, Beth. Kylie had been increasingly unhappy with the fact that Beth was soon to leave her job and she had become increasingly withdrawn over the last few days. For the last two days Kylie had sat by herself on an empty table, refusing to sit by Beth or even talk to her. Beth was pleased therefore that Kylie had now chosen to resume her seat by her side.

Without warning Kylie picked up her plate and pushed it into Beth's face. The noise ceased instantly as everyone looked up to see what would happen next. The look on Kylie's face said she knew she had gone too far. Beth let out an audible sigh and said 'Well that's lunch finished. I wonder what's for tea.' The place erupted in laughter and the tension within Kylie visibly dissipated, but before it went too far, with everyone else attempting the same thing with their neighbour, Beth turned to Kylie and invited her out of the room to talk about what she had done and her feelings about Beth leaving. As Beth and Kylie left the dining area the officer-in-charge took control and told everyone to get on with their meal.

Outside, Beth gently but firmly told Kylie that her behaviour was unacceptable and was able to discuss the reasons why the behaviour occurred.

ACTIVITY 5.10

Think through, or in a group discuss:

1 How else could this situation have been handled?

2 Have you ever used humour to manage aggression? Please describe.

3 What do you think about the use of humour to manage aggression?

12 Non-response

There are occasions when it may be appropriate not to respond directly to the behaviour. Sometimes a child, for example, has learned to gain attention by being disruptive or noisy, or by throwing things or having tantrums. Even if such behaviour had previously resulted in a smack, that smack was still attention and, for some, negative attention is the only attention received.

When the disruptive act is taking place, without ignoring the behaviour turn your attention to the other children who are responding positively and focus upon them by reassuring or working with them. Alternatively, focus upon some aspect of your work while still being aware of the child. Initially the behaviour may worsen. However, as long as the child is not in danger and not endangering others, be prepared to wait for the behaviour to abate. Once the child ceases the aggressive act, return your attention to him/her and praise him/her for ceasing. If the behaviour starts up again, once more refocus your attention elsewhere, being ready to re-praise once the behaviour has ceased.

13 Leaving

Leaving is a valid option and sometimes it is the only recourse available. How we leave a situation is important and there are a variety of ways to do this, dependent upon the circumstances facing you. You can:

- back away slowly without showing fear
- use deception, e.g.:
  'This sounds important, I'll just get my notebook'
  'I'll get us a cup of tea'
  'I'll just go and tell my manager about this'
- acknowledge the situation and arrange to meet at another time, e.g.:
  'Tempers are getting frayed. Let's take a break and get back together in ten minutes'
- walk away purposefully taking any other vulnerable people with you (if possible)
- state that you are going to leave and do so
- be called away by a colleague
- use other distraction methods (see below)
- run

ACTIVITY 5.11

In a group discuss:

In what situations is it not possible for you to leave?

Within residential and day-care units where the worker is responsible for a group of vulnerable individuals some staff feel unable to leave because of the need to protect other service users. It is imperative that agencies anticipate this and make explicit their expectations of staff, because of the possibility of conflict between workers' and service users' safety. After all, there is a rehearsed response to the fire alarm which allows everyone involved to know what they should do to evacuate the building should a fire occur. Yet frequently little thought has been given to the process of staff leaving a violent situation. Without clear procedures the implicit message given by the organisation is an expectation that staff should stay and cope, even with the most violent of situations. Yet leaving is sometimes the only option available for ensuring personal safety, and must never be ruled out.

14 Distraction

The energy of aggression is often sudden and loud and is usually accompanied by the emotion of anger. Distraction is the use of similar energy but without the emotion. Distraction may be a loud noise such as a shout or a scream, or it may be achieved by banging an object. In some instances it may be a vibration, a sudden movement or an instantaneous change of lighting. It is unexpected and shocking and can have the impact of momentarily freezing the aggressor. However, as the impact is short-lived, distraction must be accompanied by some other action(s) either to ensure personal safety or to regain control of the situation.

Personal security alarms (sometimes referred to as rape alarms) use noise as a distraction to shock the would-be assailant, allowing the potential victim to flee the scene. However, the majority of us can use our voices. A loud shout in the face of an aggressor can effectively stun the person.

Do not use this technique if the assailant has a gun or other weapon which may be triggered by an instinctive recoil action by the aggressor.

The method is most effective when close up to the aggressor and when the noise or action is loud or extreme.

CASE STUDY

The case conference was called in response to concerns over the parenting skills of Jane Donaldson, a single mother who had recently given birth to twin boys. The Health Visitor was anxious in view of Jane's age (17 years); the fact that Jane had previously been in care, and had no extended family close by; and because on the occasion of her visit the Health Visitor had found the twins crying in a pram on the landing outside Jane's flat. At that time Jane had said to the Health Visitor that she felt unable to cope with the boys.

The meeting was attended by eight people in total including Jane. It was opened by the chairperson who voiced the concerns of the Health Visitor before inviting her to bring the conference up to date. Throughout it was a difficult meeting, with Jane frequently interrupting with ranting accusations, threats and sarcastic and acerbic comments. The majority of these interruptions were ignored by the chairperson or dealt with by offering a sympathetic ear and reassuring comments.

It was when the care manager began to speak that the comments became even more personal and direct, and statements like *'you've never helped me'* and *'what do you know'* and even *'you lesbian'* were left unchallenged. Eventually the care manager turned to Jane and began to defend herself with: *'Look Jane, I tried for years to help you. But you just won't listen.'*

Whereupon Jane shot to her feet and started shouting: *'You fucking liar. You lot never did nothing for me.'*

The chairperson slammed his hand down on the desk and then quietly into the silence that followed said: *'Jane, stop shouting. Sit down and we can get this meeting over. But if you keep on shouting and making threats I'll call the police.'*

ACTIVITY 5.12

Individually consider, or in a group, discuss:

1 How else might this situation have been managed?

2 What are the pros and cons of using distraction?

3 In what situations might you use the distraction technique?

Do not overuse distraction within a residential or day-care setting as service users will become familiar with it and familiarisation with the technique diminishes its effectiveness. Overuse could also lead to you being labelled as hysterical!

For an additional example of distraction see also 'Responding to alarms', p. 65.

Unable to leave?

All of the above techniques can help to manage aggression, but they will not all work all of the time and some may be less or more effective with different people. They are designed to help ensure personal safety and/or to help regain control within a difficult situation. The LEAVING option must always be available to you because sometimes nothing else will work. However, if you are ever facing a situation where you cannot leave – where someone is pointing a gun at you, for instance:

- Stay calm.
- Breathe deeply.
- Say to yourself: 'I can get through this.'
- Make no sudden, jerky movements.
- Tell yourself you may be here for some time.
- Look around, if possible, for exits and items blocking exits.
- Sit down if you can.
- Personalise by using the word 'I' and your name if possible.
- Listen to what is being said and go along with it as far as you are able.

- If you can leave without risk, do so. The police would always prefer to have information about what is happening on the inside to help in their negotiations.

Conclusion

You are important and ensuring your personal safety is paramount. Practise these techniques so that, should you ever need them, you can call upon them. Find out which ones you feel most and least comfortable with and, if you think one or more will not work for you, do not use it. Make use of those techniques that you feel will work for you. If nothing works, do not blame yourself, because some behaviours are unmanageable.

The following activity is designed to help practise the use of defusion techniques.

ACTIVITY 5.13

Preparation prior to this exercise:
- Use three separate cards (index size) and label 1, 2 and 3.
- On card 1 write: 'OBSERVER and timekeeper. Watch the defuser for appropriate body language and listen for appropriate words used'
- On card 2 write: 'DEFUSER. Use your own method to defuse/take the heat out of the aggression'
- On card 3 write: 'AGGRESSOR. Tell of a situation where you experienced aggression. Then be prepared to play the part of the aggressor'

The exercise:
- Divide into small groups of three participants
- Give each group one set of the three cards
- On a flipchart show the following information:

  A tells of a situation where he/she faced aggression   (5 minutes)
  A and B enact the situation with C observing   (30 seconds–2 minutes max.)
  A and B say how it felt to be in role   (3–5 minutes)
  C gives feedback of B's verbal and body language and there is discussion of this feedback   (3–5 minutes)

- Pass cards clockwise and repeat the process with a different A and a different story.
- Allow 45 minutes for the enactments and ensure that each group is allocated separate rooms.

Once each participant has had the opportunity of play enactment, reconvene the large group to discuss: *What did you learn from doing this exercise?*

- Trainer to draw out information regarding defusion techniques employed, difficulty in being aggressive, difficulty in managing the aggression, value of techniques and body language employed.

KEY POINTS: PART C

By now you are aware:

☐ Aggression is unacceptable, though it may be understandable.

☐ Aggression is for the most part a behaviour that can be managed.

☐ There are a variety of techniques available to manage aggressive behaviour.

☐ Defusion techniques require both verbal and non-verbal skills.

☐ Managing aggressive behaviour is not easy for many of us and although there are techniques available these usually have to be practised.

☐ Sometimes nothing works.

☐ You are allowed to say to service users: 'Stop shouting at me.'

☐ It is acceptable to leave a situation.

☐ It is not always easy to leave a situation.

☐ Feeling responsible for another person can be dangerous.

☐ You are important and personal safety is paramount.

KEY READING

Booker, O. (1999) *Averting Aggression: Safety at Work with Adolescents and Adults*. Russell House Publishing.

Leadbetter, D. and Trewartha, R. (1999) *Handling Aggression and Violence at Work: A Training Manual*. Russell House Publishing.

Lindenfield, G. (1993; rev. edn 2000) *Managing Anger: Simple Steps to Dealing with Frustration and Threat*. Thorsons.

PART D
PHYSICAL INTERVENTIONS

In this part I want to consider the issue of physical restraint when used as a means of managing aggression. In particular I hope to address the frequently asked question, '*What can I do to protect myself, or others who may be being assaulted?*'

The use of physical measures to contain or control behaviour is always a contentious issue and one that often creates confusion, anxiety and disharmony amongst care staff. Physical restraint of any kind is often both dangerous and distressing for all parties, and must only be used either as an emergency measure to deal with a one-off situation, or within a carefully agreed and strictly monitored individual programme plan.[1] However, much physical intervention is used within social care, which may not constitute physical restraint and which may, in certain circumstances, be deemed good practice – a supportive arm around a distressed person may be an example. There is a lot of confusion about the issue of what staff are permitted to do. I have known some staff who had convinced themselves that any form of touching was prohibited, even that involved in defending themselves from an attack.

ACTIVITY 5.14

Individually make a note of some answers to the following:

(a) I think physical restraint means . . .
(b) To restrain someone is to . . .
(c) Holding is . . .

Next, in a group discuss your answers and also discuss the following:

(d) Which of the above are legal?
(e) If so, under what circumstance(s) do they become so?

In general it is a criminal offence to use physical force or to act in a way that leads another person to apprehend the use of force (for example, by raising a fist or issuing a verbal threat), unless the circumstances give rise to a 'lawful excuse' or 'justification for the use of force'.

It is also an offence to lock a person in a room without a court order, except in an emergency where, for example, the use of a locked room is a temporary measure allowing the carer to seek assistance.

Physical restraint is defined as 'the positive application of force with the intention to physically overpower the child'.[2] Although there is no specific legislation offering direct guidance about the use of physical intervention with adults, this definition may also be a useful guide in those situations (see also 'Protection for the individual', below).

Restraint may be defined as 'to prevent or hold back'. Not all forms of restraint are negative. However, those forms of restraint that coerce, force or hold a person against their will will probably be determined illegal and will require the 'lawful excuse' or 'justification for the use of force' rule.

Protection for the individual – Under law every citizen is entitled to live without interference from others, and forms of interference are recognised within both criminal and civil law. Examples of acts that may be considered unlawful include:

> False imprisonment: seclusion, confinement in a room, restricting someone to a chair, preventing, by any means, a person from leaving a room or building

> Assault: shaking a fist, throwing an object, the threatened use of a restraining device

> Battery: touching, holding, pushing, use of restrictive clothing, and even putting in a bed[3]

Physical intervention refers to the use of force to restrict movement or mobility or the use of force to disengage from dangerous or harmful physical contact initiated by the service user. Physical intervention differs from manual guidance or physical prompting in so far as it implies the use of force *against resistance*. The main difference between 'holding' and 'physical intervention' is the manner of the intervention and the degree of force applied. Physical intervention involves the application of the minimum degree of force needed to prevent injury or serious damage to property.[4]

Holding would discourage but would not in itself prevent an action.[5] With consent it is permissible, but it can still be misinterpreted and carers should therefore:

- have witnesses to the act
- not hold in unsafe environments where holding may more readily be misinterpreted, such as bedrooms, toilet, etc.
- try to avoid touching bare skin
- touch safe body zones which reduce the likelihood of arousal

In view of the emphasis on non-intervention read into the guidance provided in April 1993, and perhaps because of some of the misinterpretations placed upon the definitions used, some residential and day-care staff began to feel that the use of any form of physical contact would leave them vulnerable and open to a criminal charge. So in 1997 the Social Services Inspectorate wrote to all Directors of Social Services (see the Laming letter, p. 87) stressing the 'duty of care' element placed upon carers:

> staff and other adults responsible for children in care have, generally speaking, the same rights and responsibilities as a parent to influence the child in the interests of its welfare, to protect it from bad influences, and where necessary to protect others from harm.

In so doing the Inspectorate effectively re-emphasised the need for the use of appropriate physical interventions, without changing the fundamental message that in order to be appropriate physical intervention should:

- be deemed lawful
- only be used as a last resort
- employ the minimum reasonable force to prevent (significant) injury or avert serious damage to property

---

ACTIVITY 5.15

In a group discuss:

In what circumstances may it be reasonable to employ physical intervention?

Whilst the purpose of the guidance provided is to ensure that physical interventions are used as infrequently as possible, it is also there to ensure that when physical measures are used everything possible is done to prevent injury and maintain a person's sense of dignity. When used, examples of appropriate methods of physical intervention (dependent upon the circumstances) may include:

- two members of staff holding a service user to prevent him/her from hitting someone
- the use of specially designed equipment such as an 'arm cuff' to prevent self-injury

Inappropriate physical intervention that would be extremely difficult to justify includes:

- one or more members of staff sitting on a service user
- the use of clothing or belts to restrict movement
- holding someone face-down on the floor
- any procedure that involves pressure against joints
- any procedure that restricts breathing or impacts upon airways
- seclusion (except where the Mental Health Act 1983, or other legislation, applies)

Situations where intervention may be required and deemed appropriate are those situations that require intervention to prevent a significant risk of harm, and may, for example, include those that prevent:

- a child from running into a busy road
- self-injury
- injury to another
- serious damage to property

Emergency and planned interventions

Two situations need to be considered: (a) unplanned intervention used in an emergency, and (b) planned intervention. In either situation the general rule of only being used as a last resort to prevent serious damage applies.

ACTIVITY 5.16

Consider the following case study:

Yesterday evening Lee's mother failed to arrive for the planned visit and Nina, the assistant officer-in-charge, had spoken to Lee about this. Lee had been unhappy because he had expected sympathy from Nina and instead was told it was his aggressive behaviour towards his mother on the previous visit that had decided her against this visit.

Lee, who had been in a mood all day because of what he felt was a false accusation by Nina, spent the day creating trouble. He had refused to go to school, had 'accidentally' broken the TV remote control unit, had been surly to any and everyone, and twice had said to staff that he was going to 'get her', meaning Nina, when she came back on duty. He went out at four, returned even more angry, and tried to pick a fight with another of the lads. This had been stopped by one of the care staff, but Lee's mood worsened and once again the threat of 'just wait till the bitch gets back' was made.

Nina arrived at a few minutes before five and popped her head into the lounge, whereupon Lee picked up a pool cue and began to walk purposefully towards her.

1 If other staff were present in the lounge, would this situation call for physical intervention? If so, how?

2 If you were between Nina and Lee what would you do to protect her?

3 What could have been done to prevent this situation from occurring?

In the above case study the 'last resort' element may mean that a distraction technique should be considered – either shouting at Lee to 'stop' or at Nina to tell her to run. Maybe even grabbing hold of the cue should be attempted. However, if I were Nina, in that situation I would probably want you to do something and not be paralysed into doing nothing for fear of acting inappropriately. Section 8 of the Children's Homes Regulations 1991 states 'the taking of any action immediately necessary to prevent injury to any person, or serious damage to property' is not prohibited. It must be clear, however, that unless immediate action had been taken there were strong indicators that injury would follow.

Staff are sometimes unclear about whether they can intervene to stop a person from leaving a building. However, the guidance on this point is clear:

> where it is likely that if a young person were to leave the unit and there was a strong likelihood of injury to himself or others, it would be reasonable to use physical restraint to prevent him/her from leaving.

The British Institute of Learning Disabilities offers the following advice:

> Before using physical intervention in an emergency, the person concerned should be confident that the adverse outcomes associated with the intervention (for example injury or distress) will be less severe than the adverse consequences which would have occurred without the use of a physical intervention.[6]

Where planned intervention is considered, it should be:

- agreed in advance by a multidisciplinary team
- after consultation with the service user, their carer(s) and/or those with parental responsibility
- implemented under supervision
- carried out by staff member(s) with relevant training and experience
- reasonable
- appropriate
- included in the care plan of the service user
- recorded in writing

The continuation of such planned intervention must be regularly reviewed and must only take place as an act of care and with the intention of treatment or therapy.

KEY POINTS: PART D

☐   The use of physical interventions to control or manage behaviour is contentious.

☐   Physical intervention must be a last resort.

☐   Staff have a right to protect themselves and others.

☐   All forms of physical contact can be deemed a criminal offence.

The aim for every residential and day-care staff member must be to create an atmosphere where the use of physical intervention is not required. But where it is used, it must be used appropriately, allowing for maintenance of the person's dignity.

REFERENCES

1 Department of Health (2000) *Draft Guidance on the Use of Physical Interventions for Staff Working with Children and Adults with Learning Disability and/or Autism* (website: www.doh.gov.uk/learningdisabilities/dgapp1.htm).
2 Department of Health (1993) *Guidance on Permissible Forms of Control in Children's Residential Care* (website: www.doh.gov.uk).
3 East Sussex County Council. Social Services department. April 2000. *Restrictive Physical Interventions*.
4 See 1 above.
5 See 2 above.
6 See 1 above.

KEY READING

British Association for People with Learning Disabilities (1996) *Physical Interventions: A Policy Framework*. BILD Publications.
The Children Act (1989) Guidance and Regulations (1991) Volume 4: Residential Care. HMSO.

CHAPTER 6

BULLYING AT WORK

This chapter focuses upon the bullying of employees and considers how this form of aggression can have a devastating impact both upon the individuals concerned and upon service delivery. Besides helping to identify bullying, the chapter examines those elements that allow it to flourish. Consideration is also given to the difference between bullying and harassment at work.

The chapter identifies three different types of bullies and provides indicators to help you spot them. There is also a brief résumé of the legislative framework that may be used to beat the workplace bully.

Additionally the chapter considers the organisational responses required to eliminate bullying at work whilst also providing the person being bullied with a guide for managing it.

OBJECTIVES

By the end of this chapter you should:

▩ Have a clearer understanding of what bullying at work actually is.

▩ Be able to spot bullying.

▩ Be aware of the circumstances that allow bullying to be maintained.

▩ Know what to do if it happens to you.

Remember, however, that the bully starts off with all the advantages, and managing the workplace bully is not easy and not always possible

OVERVIEW

Bullying at work is unacceptable. It is extremely distressing, disruptive and damaging for the recipient and totally undesirable for the smooth functioning of the organisation. Unfortunately, however, it occurs more frequently than most of us would imagine. A survey carried out by UNISON in 1996 identified that two-thirds of individuals replying to the survey had either suffered or witnessed bullying at work.[1] Furthermore, a series of BBC programmes shown in 1998 indicated that over half of the workforce in England had experienced bullying in their workplace. These staggering statistics lead to a loss of revenue to the economy estimated at over two million pounds per year.[2]

More than this, however, are the costs borne by the individual on the receiving end of the bullying, which also impact upon service provision. These costs include:

- lowering of morale
- loss of belief in self and in skills
- psychological impacts such as stress, fear, anxiety, inability to concentrate, anger, hostility, etc.
- physiological impacts such as increased heart rate, sweating, shortness of breath, changes in blood pressure, headaches, ulcers, shakes, etc.
- demotivation
- poor or disturbed sleep patterns
- effects on family life and relationships
- panic attacks
- depression
- self-harm
- suicide

Individually, each of us may need skills to manage the workplace bully or the ability to protect ourselves and, although bullying is not specifically covered under health and safety legislation, good practice dictates that organisations provide appropriate policies and procedures aimed at eliminating it.

If the argument of 'good practice' fails to convince, a financial one may. Failure to ensure workplace policies and codes of practice covering bullying in the workplace can lead to heavy compensation payments. In the Scottish case of Ballantyne v. South Lanarkshire Council, for example, a social worker who was forced into early retirement by the 'outspoken and abrasive' behaviour of her boss won £66,000. In this out-of-court settlement, South Lanarkshire conceded the case, admitting that there had been shortcomings in how this worker was managed. A second example was settled in July 1999 when a former home care manager received £85,000 from Liverpool Council for stress related to being bullied.

ACTIVITY 6.1

Individually or with your colleagues, identify:

1 Are you aware of any bullying in your work?

2 What forms did it take?

3   Who was doing it and why?

4   What was the outcome?

IDENTIFYING BULLYING

Bullying is a form of violence. At work it is aggression that damages another person at a psychological rather than a physical level. One of the key elements in managing bullying lies in its identification, and that may not be easy.

CASE STUDY

I was a care manager working with older people in a residential home and I was a key worker for a number of the residents. One of my people, an old man of 74, had been becoming increasingly agitated over some days and I mentioned this to my manager. He said we'd better monitor it and to keep him informed. Anyway, on this day it was my routine to see Ted in the afternoon and as he wasn't about I went to his room. After knocking I let myself in as always, but this day Ted was in a real state. He was really agitated and was moving bits and pieces of his small pottery collection, small figures which he kept on his dressing table. I knew he wouldn't want them smashed but he'd already knocked two of them off. I walked over to him and said, 'Come on Ted, this isn't like you.' He turned and just came at me with the walking stick. He must have hit me twice before I was able to get out. Blood was running down my face. I don't remember much more. I know I was taken to hospital.

Back in work three weeks later I found out that Ted had died just a couple of days before I returned. It sounds really bad I know, but in a way I was grateful. You see I was still his key worker and would have been expected to pick up from where we left off. The next day, though, that was when it really got to me and I was having a little cry in the staff room when my manager came in. He invited me into his office to discuss things and I felt a little better but when he closed the door . . . well, he just started with, 'Look Judith, I know you're upset but, well, quite frankly your size intimidates me sometimes and so I'm not surprised it happened.' I didn't know what to do, or what to say, and before I had composed myself he said he wanted to help me with this 'little problem' and would be prepared to set up a series of meetings with me to help me to 'sort it out'.

ACTIVITY 6.2

Consider individually, or in a group discuss:

1   Was Judith being bullied?

2   What is your interpretation/definition of bullying?

3   What would you do if you were Judith's manager?

UNISON, in their campaign 'Bullying at Work'[3] describe bullying as:

> **offensive, intimidating, malicious, insulting or humiliating behaviour, abuse of power or authority which attempts to undermine an individual or group of employees and which may cause them to suffer stress.**

Examples of bullying

- shouting at individuals or groups
- humiliating individuals
- making work-life difficult for those who could do the bully's job better
- constant or unjustified negative criticism
- removing responsibility
- watching for and then pointing out mistakes
- constantly finding fault
- refusing to grant reasonable requests for leave, training, etc. without reasonable justification
- picking on individuals in front of others or in private
- imposing unreasonable or continually changing workloads or deadlines
- insisting that there is only one way to do things
- setting people up to fail by overloading them with work
- withholding information
- frequent hostile or intimidatory stares
- purposefully ignoring individuals
- unfair or discriminatory treatment

Are there occasions when doing any of the above may not constitute bullying?

HARASSMENT AND BULLYING

Harassment differs from bullying in that with harassment the perception is that there is something 'different' about the victim. This 'difference' is commonly perceived as a sexual, racial, disability or age difference. In bullying, this 'difference' is not apparent. Anyone can be subjected to bullying.

The 'bully' is often perceived as an individual who uses their weight, size and physical strength in a manner designed to intimidate another. This is indeed one form of bully and it is perhaps the more familiar image of the bully many of us meet as children. However, within the workplace the bully is more sophisticated than this. The workplace bully is an abuser of power. This may be 'real' power, as in the case of the bullying manager who, for example, may be influential over their victims' careers; 'self-perceived' power, as in the case of the long-employed bullying colleague; or 'given' power, where we allow the behaviour to continue because it is easier to ignore than to challenge. Often the workplace bully will make use of this power, bringing in subtle elements of fear, intimidation and threats which are not easy to identify. Bullying can involve negative criticism, sarcasm or even a subtle change in tone or delivery. It could be the frequent use of the 'silent stare' or the 'cold shoulder'. It could involve belittling a person, or making a person aware that their performance is being monitored and that it will not stand up to scrutiny no matter how good it is. Frequently the bully may attempt to put the 'problem' on to their victim – for example, *'Have you always had difficulty with authority?'* – then make it known to other senior figures within the agency that he/she is working with their victim to help them through this. These subtle factors make bullying difficult to spot.

Bullying is not necessarily confined to one individual.

CASE STUDY

I obtained the post of team manager within a team where the team dynamics could only be described as insular. Although there had been one or two 'outsiders' to the team over the years, most of the team were made up of people appointed from within the organisation. The outsiders, who were more vocal and who wanted to change what could only be described as outdated practice, were usually isolated and excluded and had eventually left. I had competed for the job alongside two internal applicants, neither of whom was as qualified or experienced as myself, but both of whom were presently members of the existing team.

As soon as I arrived in post my job was made extremely difficult. My competence was questioned almost daily. Statements like *'that's not the way we do it around here'* and *'it must be difficult for you adjusting to a different approach'* were commonplace from the team members. Elements of the work I had delegated were left undone and the excuses given – which were considered 'reasonable' by the rest of the team – were completely unacceptable. No one would volunteer for anything, so much so that I ended up covering the holidays and I was always the last out of the office and things like that. Getting the cases allocated was extremely difficult and getting the 'more difficult' ones allocated was a nightmare. In supervision with my line manager I was told *'things will settle down'* and *'it'll take time for them to get to know you'.* Eventually my manager had begun to suggest that he would understand if I chose to leave, and if I chose that action *'no stain'* would show on any future reference.

It eventually came to a head, however, when I found out that some of the team, with the full knowledge of the others, were actually taking my decisions to be scrutinised by the previous manager who had retired and was living nearby. I was furious, but felt so powerless, especially when I was told by my manager that he couldn't regulate who the team members contacted.

ACTIVITY 6.3

In a group discuss:

1   Was the team manager being bullied? By whom?

2 What should be done in such a situation?

3 What would you do:

   (a) if you were the team manager?

   (b) if you were a member of the team?

Currently, there is no specific legislation covering bullying at work. However, there is the opportunity to use the 'whistle blowers' legislation which was set up to get rid of abusive regimes (see Chapter 1), or harassment legislation.

Harassment legislation

Sexual and racial harassment constitute unlawful discrimination under the Sex Discrimination Act 1975 (as amended) and the Race Relations Act 1976. Harassment on the grounds of disability is not specifically defined in law. However, the Disability Discrimination Act 1996 outlaws less favourable treatment of an individual on grounds that relate to their disability. The Criminal Justice and Public Order Act 1994 makes intentional harassment a criminal offence. Although primarily intended to combat racial harassment, this legislation can be argued to be equally applicable to harassment on the grounds of sex, sexual orientation, age and disability. Furthermore there is scope for the Sex Discrimination Act being used in certain circumstances where there is sexual harassment of lesbians or gay men by heterosexuals.

The four major forms of harassment in the workplace are commonly identified as:

- **Sexual harassment** – behaviour or language of a sexual nature affecting the dignity of women or men, which is unwanted, unwelcome and unreciprocated and which may threaten job security or create a hostile, offensive or intimidating working environment for one or more employees.

- **Racial harassment** – behaviour or language towards another employee, group of employees or their property, which causes them to feel humiliated, patronised, threatened or intimidated because of their racial or ethnic origin.

- **Disability harassment** – words, actions or deeds that cause the individual worker or group of workers to be, or feel, disadvantaged, humiliated, patronised or threatened because of their capacity or capabilities.

- **Age harassment** – behaviour or language that focuses upon a person's inabilities or incapacities by virtue of their age. This may include derogatory comments and patronising behaviour and is focused around weakness and not the inherent strengths of the individual or group of workers concerned.

None of these definitions would cover the situations outlined in the two case studies so far considered in this chapter.

In your workplace do you have a policy covering 'Bullying'? Is it covered within your 'Harassment' policy? If so, does it have a separate definition?

WHO BULLIES?

In harassment the focus for the behaviour emanates from the perceived 'difference' of the person on the receiving end of the behaviour. Its foundation, its infliction and its maintenance are out of prejudice. Bullying, however, does not rely upon prejudice, though it could be a component.

ACTIVITY 6.4

In a group, with one person using a flipchart:

From your knowledge and/or experience, list any factors that may help identify the workplace bully.

Types of workplace bully

There are three types of workplace bully:

1   the person who does it out of habit
2   the person who does it under pressure
3   the person who does it to go along with others

Considering each of these in turn:

1 The person who does it out of habit

This person has done it before and they will do it again. This bully may well have started bullying in school, or may have been subjected to it. This bully functions at one of three emotional levels. He/she can:

(a)   derive much personal satisfaction from their attempts to undermine, use and damage their victim(s)
(b)   lack insight and awareness of the impact of their behaviour
(c)   simply not care about any damage being inflicted upon the individual

This bully is usually inadequate and fearful that someone else can function better or is more capable then they are at their job. They are often drawn to positions of power as a means of abusing that power. They are dictatorial and critical. They are often incompetent and are carried in their job by the very ones they bully. They will leave a trail of people in their wake who have been bullied by them, many of whom will have left the organisation. This bully is the most difficult to change.

2 The person who does it under pressure

This bully may evoke some sympathy from those around him/her because there appears to be an understandable reason for their behaviour. They are not doing it for personal satisfaction but as a means of getting the job done. They effectively become blinkered under pressure and are often themselves unaware of their behaviour. However, this bully is often hard to deal with simply because we do not know where we stand. Without the pressure this bully may well revert back to the 'nice' person we all knew and loved beforehand, but once the pressure is felt again the bullying behaviour will reappear.

The confusion for the victim created by this inconsistent approach can for some be even worse than that created by the out-and-out bully we can all identify. This type of bullying behaviour may be changed by awareness, training and close, constructive supervision.

3 The person who does it to go along with others

This person is often used as the tool of the covert bully, who may be either of the above. This bully will frequently have low self-esteem and will seek approval and support of others within 'the group'. Often becoming protective of the group they agree a set of clandestine norms, and anyone failing to adhere to these is likely to become their subject. They like the feel of being 'like-minded' and having others around them whom they identify as like-minded. They are often afraid of change and feel safer with routine and procedure.

This bully likes to perceive themselves as caring and compassionate, yet they are often hostile and critical towards the ones who in their mind 'do not fit in'. They do not want to consider the impact of their behaviour and often justify their hostility in terms of identifying the other person as being wrong or somehow deserving of this behaviour. This type of bully can be changed by breaking up the group, training, awareness and close, supportive supervision.

Profile

All too frequently the bully is someone who has done it before. In many social care organisations the bully may be well-known, often being allowed to continue their behaviour because others are afraid to challenge it. This fear is further compounded by the bully who tries to build up a protective field of individuals they consider to be of value around themselves. Not infrequently the bully will ally themselves with powerful people or decision makers within or associated with the organisation. Part of the reason behind this is an attempt to make them and their behaviour invulnerable to criticism or change, and as this web of individuals may include the union representative, the assistant director, or director, the bully's invulnerability seems assured.

The bully may have used charm to worm their way into the awareness of these 'key players', or they may have made themselves appear invaluable to the individual by providing useful information. They may seek also to ally themselves with 'powerful' individuals outside of, but who hold influence over, the organisation, such as local dignitaries or officials.

Another device used by some bullies is the systematic and cynical use of sexual liaisons with fellow workers. The bully will engage in sexual liaison at one of two levels within the organisation:

(a)   at a senior level in order to compound their invulnerability
(b)   with subordinate staff as a means of gaining information about the mood of the staff force in general and about any dissent from individuals in particular

Such liaison allows the bully to take pre-emptive moves to ward off any actions proposed against them.

Does anyone in your organisation match the above profile?

Other factors

Unfortunately the above profile can also match innocent individuals who are committed to furthering the needs of the organisation. However, the difference lies in the fact that the bully is furthering their own needs at the expense of the organisation, and that factor can often be identified if looked for.

- Bullies lie, often misrepresenting information exchanged during their encounters with their victims – this can be an identified pattern occurring in different workplaces and involving different victims.
- Many have been the subject of disciplinary hearings which have found the case against them unproven or unsubstantiated because of a lack of tangible evidence.
- They often leave behind them a trail of subordinates who have moved position because of stress, or who have left the job for unaccountable reasons, undeclared personal reasons or ill-health.
- Stress levels in staff subordinate to the bully are often higher than normal.
- Staff are often aware of the bully from interactions with other staff.
- Many bullies are promoted away from the service users because their practice is deemed to be faulty or even dangerous, and they are moved as a means of preventing harm. This provides them with a greater influence over a larger number of workers.
- Bullies prefer to do their bullying in private away from the public glare.
- They can be charming in front of 'outsiders'.[4]

Are you aware of anyone within your organisation who bullies staff?

How do they get away with it?

Sometimes, the person who is the bully may be the most powerful person within the organisation.

CASE STUDY

Dave was a first line manager in charge of a team of social workers and had been in this post for over six years. At this time the agency began to experience major changes to the way it delivered services to the public. The changes were designed to save money but the draconian way they were brought into action created many problems. A new director had been appointed and communication through the department, once easy and clear, was now done in memo form only.

Staff morale was low and people were constantly in fear of 'getting it wrong'. Team meetings and supervision sessions were reduced, service provision was prioritised, and suddenly Dave's team began to become the target of anger from other professionals as well as service users.

Dave was committed to the service and enjoyed his job which was now becoming increasingly stressful. The final straw, however, was when senior management decreed that a number of middle management positions had to go. Team managers were all informed they would have their current contracts terminated and they would have to reapply for a new position within the new structure which contained six fewer team manager posts. Rumour and conjecture, about who would get the new posts and who would not, were rife, and coincidentally information was passed from senior management that the best jobs would go in the first round. There was also a time limit of three months placed upon implementation of the new structure. In order to get the best jobs, or in fact keep their own, team managers therefore had to get their new contracts signed and their applications in within two weeks.

Dave decided, for whatever reason, that this was wrong. He simply refused to sign away his old contract or apply for a new one.

First, Dave was contacted by an Assistant Director whom he had not seen for over twelve months. Over a series of telephone calls a lot of emotive pressure was applied, from 'Come on Dave, you know how valued you are, you can't let us down like this' and 'Don't you think it's strange no one else is taking this stance', to 'If you're worried about not being able to manage the new job, you don't have to you know.' Ultimately the Assistant Director called to see Dave in his office and told him 'It's out of my hands now, there's nothing more I can do for you.'

After a week Dave received a telephone call from the Director's secretary, inviting him to a meeting with the Director to discuss 'any fears about the new structure'.

At the meeting, which Dave attended unaccompanied, Dave was threatened with the loss of his job, he was told he would never work again in social work, and he was given one hour in which to change his mind and sign the contract which the Director threw at him. Dave refused and after leaving the Director's office managed to hold on to his tears until he was alone.

Dave instigated disciplinary procedure against his Director. During the intervening months while awaiting the hearings, Dave's team was dispersed throughout the agency, his original supportive line manager was replaced by a less supportive one, and Dave's duties were substantially altered – he was given the responsibility of ensuring the filing was done correctly. He was also made to sign in and out, and the case files on which Dave had been working were taken to head office for 'examination'.

The disciplinary hearings were all chaired by Dave's Director and after nine months the conclusion of the procedure found 'no case' to answer. Dave then appealed to the local council, and upon having proven his case he was made redundant and provided with the minimum legal redundancy payment permissible.

ACTIVITY 6.5

As a group:

1 Describe the arena in which behaviour like this can flourish.

2 Identify any similarities to your workplace.

Bullying is more likely to occur in workplaces which have:

- management by fear or an authoritarian management
- an absent, hierarchical management
- an over-competitive atmosphere
- fears of redundancy
- fears of loss of status
- envy and jealousy amongst staff
- poor communication where gossip and rumour are rife
- excessive workloads and demands on people
- impossible targets and/or deadlines to meet
- a culture of seeking to blame rather than to learn
- lack of training opportunities
- little participation
- scapegoating

ACTIVITY 6.6

Individually or in a group identify:

1 Which of the above elements occur within your workplace?

2 What can be done to:

   (a) change these?
   (b) ensure they do not occur?

SO WHAT CAN BE DONE?

Organisational responses

In the second case study (see p. 122), clearly the line manager had a role to play in helping the team manager to function appropriately.

The line manager, as part of the senior departmental management team, could:

- actively promote a working environment in which bullying is viewed as unacceptable

- actively identify bullying for what it is and make clear statements about acceptable and unacceptable ways of behaving
- raise staff awareness regarding their responsibilities and codes of conduct towards fellow members of staff
- actively promote an environment in which staff feel able to challenge bullying
- tackle situations at a low level before they escalate
- gather information and/or evidence
- take immediate action to investigate situations
- set standards of behaviour which actively demonstrate the above principles
- ensure that a formal anti-bullying policy is in place

ACTIVITY 6.7

In a group, brainstorm:

The elements contained within an anti-bullying policy should include . . .

Some organisations have established Harassment Officers with the responsibility to provide advice and support to those making contact. Their role can be either formal or informal and is strictly confidential. The Harassment Officer is able to offer advice about the policy of the agency. Some Harassment Officers are charged with collecting and collating information about bullying as a means of helping to identify who the bully is.

Additionally, organisations now have the power to establish an 'authorised person' under the Public Interest Disclosure Act 1998 (see Chapter 1). One of the powers of this officer could be to investigate situations of bullying where, for example, the situation might lead to a danger to the health of the employee.

Under the Public Interest Disclosure Act, who is your authorised officer?

Individual action

Do not make the mistake of thinking that it will be easy to manage the workplace bully. It is often extremely difficult, especially in organisations that do not have a specific anti-bullying policy. Policies often provide those subjected to bullying with a constructive framework as well as the knowledge that they are not alone.

It is extremely daunting for an individual to try to deal with a bully who is a part of the structure of the organisation, as it often takes on the David and Goliath quality of a lone individual pitted against the might of an organisation. This is particularly pertinent when, as identified, one of the ploys of the bully is to ally themselves with key players within the organisation.

The feeling of powerlessness is common. Indeed it is often one of the aims of the bully to bring about this perception within their victim. In fact, there are a number of actions and choices open to anyone who is being bullied. The following action plan is a list of suggestions which may help to regain some control over a situation.

ACTIVITY 6.8

Individually consider, or in a group, identify:

1 What would be your feelings if you were being bullied at work?

2 What would you do if you were being bullied at work?

3 What would you do for a colleague who was being bullied at work?

Action plan

1 **First of all ACKNOWLEDGE that you may be being bullied**. This may not be as easy as it initially appears. Many of us may not like to acknowledge that we are the one who is being bullied, mistakenly thinking that only certain people – those with a 'victim mentality' – are the subject of the workplace bully. Sometimes we try to work harder in an attempt to please or placate the bully – to, in effect, try to put things right. We may feel it is somehow our fault, especially if other people around us are not receiving the same sort of treatment. As a consequence, self-image can suffer, we begin to feel less capable or competent in our work and this can then have the effect of confirming the bully's actions.

2 **KEEP NOTES** of everything with DATES and TIMES. A pattern of incidents helps to confirm that it is not happening by chance. Note down everyday criticisms; the repeated unrealistic demands; the constant notification that your colleagues are better than you; the repeated questions about your commitment, ability and skills; the exclusions from the team get-togethers; the failure to be given up-to-date information; the excuses used for forgetting to notify you of that meeting; the times when you are set up to fail by being given those impossible jobs to complete in totally unrealistic time scales; or the occasions when you are given those tasks way below your status or level of ability. All can build up into a picture of being bullied, and when documented will help you to identify that you are not over-reacting.

3 **KEEP EVIDENCE.** Sometimes scribbled notes may be left on your work. Your work may be returned with crossings-out, or even the 'accidental' spilt tea over it, or even the popular 'DO AGAIN' without any explanation of what is wrong with it. Anonymous notes may be left on your desk.

   You may be shouted at or criticised in front of your work colleagues and have the evidence of witnesses.

4 **HAVE WITNESSES.** Try not to be alone with the bully, and make a note of anyone who may have witnessed the behaviour. Be aware, however, that often other colleagues do not want to become involved because they are afraid of losing their job, concerned that the bully may turn upon them or, if they are unaware of the bullying, they may not want to take sides.

5   Try using **ASSERTIVE RESPONSES** (see Chapter 5). Often it is the bully who takes the lead, and frequently those being bullied are reacting to the situation rather than taking some control over it themselves. Practise with a friend or family member what you are going to say, should it happen again. Learning how to say 'No' effectively or learning how to respond to negative criticism without becoming hostile can help to bring a feeling of some power over the situation. Sometimes if the bully is stood up to in an assertive manner the bullying stops.

6   Taking **TIME OFF** can prove an invaluable way of giving you time to think things through calmly. It can help to rethink a situation or plan, help to regenerate ideas on how to manage the situation, or even allow you to decide whether or not you want to stay. If you do not want to take sick leave, why not take time off by going on a training course – on learning how to be assertive, for example? This will give you time out, help you to formulate some strategies, and help you to find out what the job is like in other agencies or within other departments.

7   **DO NOT SUFFER IN SILENCE.** If you can talk it over with a senior member in your department or office, do so, but choose carefully. Talking it over with friends and colleagues can really help and it may bring in allies, as the bully may also be intimidating someone else within the agency. Besides helping to 'get it off your chest', letting others know what is happening to you can be productive, as bullies like to do their bullying away from the public glare, and the more talk about their activities the less happy they are.

8   Use the agency's **POLICIES** on **BULLYING** or **HARASSMENT**, or the agency's **COMPLAINTS PROCEDURE**. Increasingly agencies are becoming aware of this as a real issue and a significant number are providing policy statements covering this area of staff support. Many agencies are providing Harassment Officers for staff to approach formally or informally. Using the agency's complaints procedure is daunting and will take a lot of time and consequently much emotional energy, but it can be successful. Remember the 'Whistle blowing' legislation (Chapter 1), and if your agency has an 'approved person' to approach consider doing this.

9   Involve your **UNION**. Think seriously about joining one if you are not already a member. It can be easy to feel isolated and powerless, especially in the situation where the bully may be your boss. Find out what the union is doing about the issue. If you do use the complaints procedure it is often less isolating to be accompanied by a union representative to any meetings this may involve.

10 Your agency has a 'duty to care' and if it fails in this it can be deemed liable, so you may have recourse to **LEGAL ACTION** against your employer, or you may wish to seek redress via an Industrial Tribunal. This is not an easy option and although a number of high-profile cases have resulted in substantial awards being paid to employees I wonder how many more have failed. Talk it over with a union representative or solicitor. Some firms of solicitors offer a 'no win – no fee' form of representation (but look at the small print as you may have to pay for letters sent, telephone calls made and so on).

11 It may be necessary to consider another approach: **LEAVE**. It may not be possible but, if you can, leaving may provide a solution to your situation. You are important and making sure that you are OK is the important thing. Often the

next company or organisation can have a completely different culture. If you do choose to leave, make sure that you feel all right about the action by praising yourself for doing something about it – after all, strategic withdrawal is a recognised valid tactic. All too often, however, we will feel a failure, even when we have tried every approach. Remember, sometimes nothing works and leaving is the only option left.

12   Finally, whatever you choose to do about the situation, always **GIVE YOURSELF THE APPROPRIATE PRAISE** for your actions.

KEY POINTS

By now you are aware of:

☐   How to spot the workplace bully.

☐   The effects it can have upon the individual, and the costs of bullying to the organisation.

☐   The arena in which bullying can flourish.

☐   Three types of bully.

☐   The organisational response required to help eliminate it.

☐   An individual action plan to help manage it.

Bullying at work is unacceptable and in this chapter I hope to have provided you with a few ideas to help to get rid of the workplace bully.

REFERENCES

1   'Bullying at Work' – survey report carried out on behalf of UNISON by Staffordshire University Business School in 1998. Published as a web page on: www.workdoctor.com/home/twd/employers/unison.html
2   BBC Education. Series of programmes shown on TV in 1998. BBC Education – *Bullying: A Survival Guide*. Information from: www.bbc.co.uk/education/archive/bully/
3   UNISON campaign: 'Bullying at Work'. Details from: www.unison.org.uk/
4   Field, T. (1996) *Bully in Sight*. Success Unlimited.

KEY READING

Clifton, J. and Serdar, H. (2000) *Bully Off! Recognising and Tackling Workplace Bullying*. Russell House Publishing.
Pollard, J. 'Please sir, you're a bully.' Article in *The Observer* newspaper, 2 April 2000.
Thompson, N. (1999) *Tackling Bullying and Harassment in the Workplace*. Pepar Publications.

INFORMATION

GPMU Campaign: 'Bullying – spotting the signs'
(website: www.gpmu.org.uk/bullysign.html).

Bully on line is an excellent website with lots of information provided by Tim Field and can be found at: www.successunlimited.co.uk/policy.htm

University of Exeter: 'Policy on the protection of dignity at work and study'. This policy statement is available to be viewed at: www.ex.ac.uk/EAD/personnel/ppdws.htm

Andrea Adams Trust is a UK national charity devoted to raising awareness of tackling bullying. Andrea Adams Trust, Maritime House, Basin Road North, Portslade, Brighton, East Sussex BN41 1WA (Tel: 01273 704900), email: aat@btinternet.com

CHAPTER 7

ETHNIC AND GENDER ISSUES

In this chapter I want to focus upon ethnic and gender issues pertinent to violence in social care. These additional factors can have a direct influence upon levels of aggression and if they are addressed appropriately the number of violent incidents faced by many social care staff can be reduced.

By focusing upon individual experiences via a number of case studies, the chapter provides additional useful general points of information in order to help identify difference, counter misconception and reduce prejudice.

OBJECTIVES

By the end of this chapter the reader should be aware of:

▨ Commonly held misconceptions about ethnic and cultural issues.

▨ Some of the ethnic considerations that social care organisations need to address.

▨ Some myths and stereotypes, and actions taken based upon these.

▨ Some impacts of gender within aggression.

ETHNIC/CULTURAL ISSUES

Within social care, black, Asian and mixed-race care staff can often experience racism which is left unchallenged by management.

CASE STUDY

Beatrice works in Horton House, a residential home for older people, and has worked there since 1989. Over the years the function of Horton House has changed as gradually the majority of residents have become increasingly infirm. The top floor of the house was redesigned as an EMI (Elderly Mentally Infirm) unit a few years ago, and all the staff are on a rota to spend some time each week working on the top floor. Beatrice does not consider the residents on the top floor as her clients and dislikes having to do her weekly shift up there. But, as she explains, 'I just get on with it and do what they [the managers] tell me.' Beatrice earns just above the minimum wage and needs her job to supplement the family income. She has received no special training in managing people with senile dementia or in the needs of older people. She was employed because of her firm desire to help.

The only training course on communication skills Beatrice has attended was one entitled 'Managing Aggression at Work', which she attended because of the increasing number of incidents experienced by her. On this training course, when asked if she had ever experienced violence at work Beatrice answered 'No', because, 'it never comes from my clients. They are really nice people. It only comes from the ones upstairs and that's the way it is for everyone.' The top-floor unit accommodates fourteen residents and usually has between two and four staff members working there at any one time. The door of the unit is kept permanently locked for fear of the residents wandering.

The type of violence she experiences from 'upstairs' includes biting, scratching, pinching, hair pulling and verbal abuse. In addition to being sworn at regularly, the major form of verbal abuse is usually racist and includes 'keep those filthy black hands off me', 'black bitch' and 'go back to your own country'. Beatrice has been told that this behaviour is because the clients suffer from dementia and that it cannot be helped.

ACTIVITY 7.1

In a group discuss:

What can be done to address this situation and bring a stop to this racism?

The above case study raises at least four elements of concern:

1   lack of appropriate staff training in basic care issues
2   staffing ratios
3   locking-up service users
4   institutionalised racism where racist comments made by service users appear to be accepted by the organisation

Institutional racism is the use or expression of racist statements or beliefs within an organisation, which remain unchallenged.

It follows, therefore, that racist behaviour:

- is expected to be tolerated by those on the receiving end
- is often excused by those in positions of authority within the organisation as the result of circumstance, e.g. 'It's not his fault, it's because he has dementia'
- may occur when the perceived needs of the client dominate a situation
- may be historical and is therefore given the status of being acceptable, e.g. 'He/she's always said that'
- is minimised, e.g. 'He doesn't mean anything by it'
- is often considered as something that the receiver must learn to deal with, and it is regarded as an inadequacy on their part if they fail to do so, e.g. 'You've just got to learn to ignore it'
- is considered as acceptable behaviour by decision makers within the organisation

The definition of institutional racism arising from the Macpherson Report[1] is:

> the collective failure of an organisation to provide an appropriate and professional service to people because of their colour, culture or ethnic origin. It can be seen or detected in processes, attitudes and behaviour which amount to discrimination through unwitting prejudice, ignorance, thoughtlessness, and racist stereotyping which disadvantage minority ethnic people.

Ethnicity is belonging to, identifying with or deriving from a group or culture usually associated with a country, continent or nation.

Prejudice is not the same as preference. Prejudice implies a negative evaluation of another person on the basis of some general attribute (such as sex, race or disability). Thus racial prejudice means a negative evaluation of people as a consequence of their being in a certain racial or ethnic group.[2]

Racial discrimination is the treatment of individuals unfavourably compared to others on the grounds of their race.

Racism is a combination of at least three elements:[3]

1 Individual racism: the basic belief that some people are subhuman and that this subhuman quality is determined by inherited biological factors such as colour of skin.
2 Institutional racism: see above.
3 Cultural racism: the values, beliefs and ideas usually embedded in our 'common sense' which endorse the superiority of one culture over others.[4]

Overview

The term 'Asian' is a cover-all term usually applied to a wide range of individuals with ethnic origins ranging from India and Pakistan to China, Indonesia, Japan and other parts of Asia. Similarly the term 'black' incorporates an enormous range of different individuals whose origins can mostly be traced to the immense continent of Africa.

This oversimplification fails to take into account the historical perspective which demonstrates that groups of individuals moving into other lands added to and derived elements from the pre-existing cultures within those lands. This may be recognised in some of the terms used to describe ethnic background today, e.g. Afro-Caribbean.

Whilst it is generally held that the two terms 'Asian' and 'black' are acceptable ways to describe an individual's ethnicity (always taking into account the person's preferences), the use of the term 'coloured' is generally to be avoided, as it is pejorative and considered offensive by many.

Many Asian, black and mixed-race people have parents and grandparents who were born in Britain. They are British, and many have adapted to the British culture, whilst others retain their own cultural norms. Some people have adopted parts of the British culture, whilst others have had it forced upon them. Some children have grown away from the traditional norms, while others assert their rights to retain their cultural identity. This is just one element of the diversity that makes up the Britain of today. Diversity adds to the wealth of a nation as it allows growth and encourages change. It is stimulating and challenging, vibrant and exciting. It also creates fear amongst some and provokes hostility within others.

ACTIVITY 7.2

Either individually or in a multicultural group, without being pejorative, identify:

1   What cultural differences are you aware of?

2   Where does your information come from?

3   How does this knowledge affect your practice?

Fighting prejudice

The Race Relations Act was passed in 1976 in an attempt to strengthen the law relating to racial discrimination. This Act sought to make acts of racial discrimination illegal. The Act also established the Commission for Racial Equality (CRE) which was established to work towards the elimination of racial discrimination and the promotion of equality of opportunity between people of different racial groups.[5]

Since this time it is interesting to consider how the offensive and degrading word 'nigger' has to all intents and purposes been dropped from the English language, even by those suffering from such illnesses as dementia.

Unfortunately, some firmly-held traditional beliefs provide additional difficulty in tackling racism. Take, for example, the belief that 'An Englishman's home is his castle' and the implicit sentiment that what goes on behind those closed doors is somehow more acceptable. This concept becomes especially pertinent in those situations where care staff are employed to work within the service user's home.

CASE STUDY

Judy is a member of the domiciliary care team and explains why she prefers to work with white colleagues when visiting one service user:

'Everybody knows Elizabeth. She's always been offensive to everyone who goes in to do for her. That's why we're all on a rota and only have to go in one week in every three. She's especially offensive towards black staff and I must admit it gets to me whenever I am asked to team up with a non-white colleague. It's not just the words, it's the gestures and noises she makes and then there's the mess. She will always soil herself whenever there is a black or Asian worker in the home. She doesn't seem to do it with the rest of us. It's like a pattern. You can always guarantee if there's a black carer then Elizabeth will mess herself. I've told them in the office that she's doing it on purpose and all they say is, "we've not got enough staff to send out two white workers all the time". Then they say it would be racist if we only sent in white workers. So I say, let's not send anyone in at all, but apparently we must go in because she's got to be looked after. But you know, something has got to be done. We've had people regularly in tears and leaving.'

ACTIVITY 7.3

Think through, or in a group, discuss:

1 Is it racist to only allocate white staff to such a situation?

2 How else may this situation be managed?

The arguments often used for allowing such situations to continue include:

1   no evidence – often it is the word of the service user against that of the worker
2   we cannot stop it from happening in their own home
3   health and safety legislation does not apply in a service user's home
4   powerlessness – there is no way of preventing it
5   we have an obligation to provide the service

Each of the above arguments can be countered:

1   evidence can be accumulated in the form of Incident Report Forms completed by different staff
2   when providing a service, contractual expectations can be established, e.g. I agree to clean your home if you agree not to be abusive or offensive in return'
3   health and safety legislation is applicable in agencies employing five or more staff, irrespective of where the staff are employed
4   appropriate sanctions can be used – these may include the withdrawal of the service temporarily or in some cases even permanently

5   Legal obligations give the agency the opportunity of returning to the court and arguing an inability to maintain service provision in its present form for fear of staff safety.

Managerial responses

The responsibility of the manager in ensuring that staff are not faced with racism is clear: because it is illegal and unacceptable it should not be tolerated. Unfortunately, as the majority of managers within social care are white[6] and middle-class, the experience of racism faced by this powerful group is negligible. If racism *was* experienced by this group I am convinced that proactive strategies would be employed to eradicate it. In the current situation, however, many white managers within social care can be accused of either purposefully or unthinkingly being:

- Colour-blind: making the assumption that all staff irrespective of their ethnic background can provide a service to all service users, thereby failing to take into account elements like xenophobia, white supremacism, hate and intolerance.
- Ignorant of the issue: failing to make the connection between abusive language and racist language.
- In search of an easy ride: knowing that racism experienced by their staff is unacceptable but choosing to do nothing about it.
- Insensitive: expecting the worker to put up with it and not to take it personally.
- Patronising: helping their worker to put up with it by supporting them through it.

The current situation is unlikely to change in the near future, especially as the number of top managers from ethnic minorities within social care is declining. Ten years ago there were five social services directors from ethnic minority backgrounds, but by the beginning of the twenty-first century there was just one.[7]

ACTIVITY 7.4

In a group identify:

What could be done by a manager to ensure that racist comments towards staff are either eradicated or reduced?

Currently some solutions may appear drastic, may be unnecessary and may be unproductive. Consider the following example:

CASE STUDY

Eve wants to maintain her daily routine of walking to the lounge after lunch. Unfortunately her condition has deteriorated so badly that she now requires the use of a walking frame. Yesterday she frightened herself when she fell, and today Manjeet has been asked by her manager to assist Eve if appropriate. Eve has previously refused offers of assistance from other Asian workers in the home but is quite happy to be assisted by the white care staff.

Eve is disgruntled and has told Manjeet to go away, that she can manage on her own, and Manjeet is now keeping a discreet eye on her while occupying herself clearing away the lunch dishes.

Eve very unsteadily manages to pull herself into the walking frame but begins to wobble and is dangerously close to overbalancing. Manjeet rushes over and is just in time to steady her with an arm around the shoulders, stopping a certain fall. 'Keep your filthy hands to yourself', shouts Eve. 'I don't need assistance from *your* kind!'

Manjeet's manager is passing and, upon hearing this, requests Eve to apologise to Manjeet. Eve refuses and re-emphasises 'I don't need help from them.'

'That's your choice', says the manager, 'but you need help to get to the lounge and Manjeet is here for that. But I won't let her help you unless you apologise.'

Eve still refuses so the manager turns to Manjeet and in Eve's hearing says 'Help her if she apologises. If she doesn't, when she falls call an ambulance.' The manager then walks off.

ACTIVITY 7.5

In a group:

Discuss the pros and cons of the action taken by Manjeet's manager.

What would you do if you were the manager?

Arguments in favour of the above approach	**Arguments against** the above approach
1 It is supportive of the staff group as it is a clear message given by the manager to the staff member that racist statements are not acceptable.	1 It is potentially punitive – if carried out the service user could fall and be injured. It therefore replaces one form of violence with another.
2 It is also a clear message to the service user that her language and/or behaviour will not be tolerated.	2 If the service user falls, it places an extra call upon scarce resources, i.e. ambulance and hospitalisation.
3 It establishes a precedent/example to other service users that this language/behaviour is unacceptable.	3 It is potentially escalatory and provocative and may force the service user into non-compliance in order to save face.

4 It re-establishes any contractual obligation on the part of the service user to treat staff with dignity and respect when being shown the same.

5 It is one way of stamping out racist statements within this establishment.

4 It creates ill will in the mind of the subject and fear in the minds of other service users.

5 It reduces the possibility of open discussion of difference and the roots of prejudice, and denies the opportunity of truly eliminating racism.

ACTIVITY 7.6

Individually consider, or in a group identify:

1 What would you do if you witnessed a colleague being verbally abused?

2 What would you do if you witnessed a colleague being racially abused?

A strategy

A lot more can be done to ensure that staff from ethnic minorities are protected, including:

1 **A clear contractual agreement**
Within social care, contracts are often provided to service users. Indeed a contract is one way of establishing the boundaries for service provision. Wherever possible these contracts should include the conditions pertinent to behaviour within which the service may be provided, amended or withdrawn. One stipulation prior to service provision would be to include a statement that racism of any sort is unacceptable and that the service will be withdrawn if such behaviour is identified.

2 **Risk assessment**
Some individuals are racist and the contractual approach may not work, yet the organisation concerned may feel obliged to provide a service. To ensure that such situations are considered, prior to intervention part of the risk assessment process (see Chapter 3) should be specifically designed to assess the safety of ethnic minority workers within the family being visited or the environment within which the worker is expected to operate, even just walking through.

3 **Discussion and information**
Within residential and day-care units there is a golden opportunity for open discussion of difference and the provision of information. Open discussion helps to dispel myth and misconception amongst both staff and service users but could arouse much ill feeling if handled inappropriately.

4   **Private discussion/affirmation**
     Where passionate feelings are aroused or expressed, a discussion of these feelings
     in private can often be more productive than in an open session where it is all too
     easy to reconfirm prejudice by stereotyping and identifying negatives.

ACTIVITY 7.7

In a group discuss:

If they come to live in this country they should do what we do.

---

5   **Positive images**
     Examples of difference displayed in posters, notices and pictures can help to
     inform.

6   **Diverse examples**
     Diversity of examples includes food, dance, religion, music, dress and festivals.
     In a residential setting it may be possible to have a Lebanese or a Caribbean
     evening, for example. Similarly visits could be arranged to local places of interest
     including places of worship.

7   **Experience of difference**
     Links could be sought with local ethnic minority groups and exchange visits
     arranged. Staff could be involved in temporary job-swaps, and some service users
     could be provided with work experience amongst minority groups.

8   **Education**
     The giving and receiving of information about ethnic or cultural difference help
     to reduce prejudice by demystifying it. It is especially productive to identify the
     elements that in the past have given rise to mythology and reaffirmed prejudice.
     Staff training in anti-racist and anti-discriminatory practice is particularly
     important, especially as many staff will not have had the opportunity to consider
     these elements before.

ACTIVITY 7.8

Make an individual list, or in a group identify:

What do you do in your workplace to help eradicate racism?

GENDER ISSUES

The following examples of research help both to confirm and to shake some of the
preconceptions we may hold about violence and gender.

- First, information from the Economic and Research Council is interesting as it appears to dispel the myth held by many that male service users are less likely to attack female service providers:

    The patterns explored here show that the various forms of violence are different for different people. Women are most likely to be physically and sexually assaulted by men. Men are most likely to be physically and sexually assaulted by other men.[8]

- Secondly, research completed by Jan Pahl provides confirmation that male staff may find themselves in a more confrontational position more frequently than their female counterparts:

    To what extent did gender, age or ethnicity make a person more vulnerable to physical attack and abuse? We carried out a series of analyses to examine the extent to which these factors were related to the experience of violence, threats of violence or verbal abuse over the last twelve months. The results showed that in general men were more likely than women to have experienced all the different types of violence. . . . A fifth of men had experienced physical attack, compared with a tenth of women.[9]

- Countering this, however, research currently being undertaken at Hertfordshire University indicates that female care staff are more likely to be on the receiving end of aggression than male care staff, although the study does concede that this may be due to the fact that care work attracts a disproportionate number of women.[10]

If, as it seems, gender does play its part in the management of aggression, it may be useful to consider specific responses based solely upon gender in order to learn from these. In an attempt to identify different responses based solely upon gender, in my training I use various case studies with a number of single-gender and mixed-gender groups. Each group is asked how they would respond to the following set of circumstances:

William is a child of 8 years and today you are responsible for his care. You have taken him out to a local play area and sit on the bench while William plays on the swings. After a while you offer him a packet of crisps which he takes to eat by the slide, a distance of about 25 metres from where you are seated. You return to reading your newspaper and fail to notice a group of 5 other children approaching William. When you look up, you see that William is surrounded by this group. One of the group is trying to take his packet of crisps while the others appear to be teasing him. He is becoming distressed and tearful. Suddenly, one of the children seizes the crisp packet, throws it to the floor and stamps on it.

What would you do now, how and why, if the group of children are:

(a) aged about 8 to 10 years?
(b) aged about 10 to 12 years?
(c) aged about 12 to 14 years?
(d) aged about 14 to 16 years?

ACTIVITY 7.9

In a mixed-gender group:

1 Identify what you would do in the above circumstances.

2 Consider any gender differences in managing this situation.

Summary of responses from all-male group	**Summary of responses from all-female group**
(a) Approach the group and ask what on earth they think they are doing. Then tell them to move on.	(a) Maybe shout first, then approach and tell the group they are behaving badly, before removing William or asking them to leave.
(b) Maybe shout, telling them to leave him alone, but definitely get to William and remove him if they would not go.	(b) Call William's name. Approach, comfort him and ask the group to consider the harm they are doing to him, before removing him.
(c) Again shout at them something like 'Oi you lot leave him alone', go over and then tell them to be on their way.	(c) A little harder because of their age and number. Would be concerned for William but probably not afraid. Would want to help William, possibly by shouting and asking him to come to me. Would explain to William afterwards that what the group was doing was wrong.
(d) Depends on their size and if other people are around. Maybe shout 'leave him alone' and see what happened next. Be prepared to get in there.	(d) Probably the same as in (c) but maybe now would be afraid. Possibly stay where I was initially. If William could not leave, would walk over briskly and take him away, focusing upon him and not the group.

I also ask groups to consider the following:

CASE STUDY

It is a dark November evening. You have called to see Mr Leith, a 90-year-old man who lives alone in a ground-floor flat on a high-rise estate. You have left your car parked by security bollards about 400 metres away. You are now walking around one of the high-rise buildings when you immediately see a group of seven older teenaged boys and girls, kicking and banging Mr Leith's door. They are shouting 'Pervert. You dirty perv.' The noise and energy levels are increasing. The youths have obviously been drinking and smashed bottles litter the doorstep.

You know that Mr Leith has never been accused of any acts of indecency. He is a very timid man who would be mortified to be accused of any wrongdoing. You also know he would be terrified in his flat with the banging and shouting. Suddenly, one of the group sees you and shouts 'There's that bastard from the council that put him here let's get 'em.' Three of the youths turn and start to walk towards you.

ACTIVITY 7.10

In a mixed-gender group identify:

1 What would you do next, how and why?

2 Are there any gender differences to the way this would be handled?

3 Would this be easier to manage if the youths were all male? Or all female?

Although the issue of personal safety should be the overriding one here, in many training situations a significant number of women – more than their male counterparts – have identified that the need to protect and ensure the safety of their client can dominate such situations. When this occurs it causes them to put their own personal safety to one side and, instead of leaving the situation to get help, they may choose to stay and attempt to negotiate with the aggressor(s).

The following case study has provided a number of similar gender-different responses.

CASE STUDY

You are working in a residential unit which is providing accommodation for young people who have been in the care of the local authority. Jake Miles, one of the longer-standing residents, who has experienced physical abuse both in his own home and whilst in care, returned a few minutes ago in a distressed state and went straight up to his room. You went up to see him but he would not let you in. You are half-way down the stairs when you see a man you do not know storm in through the front door. 'Where's the bastard', he shouts. 'I'll fucking do him.' He moves to the foot of the stairs, looks up at you and says 'I mean it and you won't stop me.' He starts to climb the stairs.

What would you do next?

Typical male responses	Typical female responses
Tell the guy to stay where he is and to stop shouting	Tell Jake to lock his door
Stay where I was as I'm in the powerful position	Sit down and talk quietly with the man, trying to calm him down
Tell him to leave or I'll call the police	Tell him I'm not going to stop him but ask him to rethink his actions. Maybe reminding him that the police could be called

From the reactions given to these case studies by the majority of participants, my personal belief is that generally within a social care setting:

Women:
* are better negotiators than men
* discuss more readily
* have a more keenly developed protective instinct and may be more readily influenced by this
* talk more freely about and are more able to express fears and anxieties

Men:
* are more confrontational and challenging
* tend to the belief that they should be able to manage a situation
* are more likely to intervene inappropriately
* are less able to express fear about a situation
* are more likely to fear losing face and therefore may stay longer within aggressive situations

Implications for practice

1   male managers may contribute to the 'macho', *it's a part of the job* culture prevalent within many social care settings
2   lack of support often experienced by staff may be a consequence of the male attitude – *you should be able to cope*
3   female staff may feel obliged to adapt to the male 'coping' culture in order to ensure progression, which in turn confirms the negative culture
4   as the majority of basic-grade workers are female, many can feel disenfranchised and powerless to effect change in a culture dominated by male attitudes
5   female staff may be more likely to confuse their 'nurturing' role, leading to the belief that behaviour should be understood at all times, therefore failing to identify it as simply *unacceptable*
6   the automatic use of male staff being called in and expected to have the ability to deal with the aggressive service user must be questioned
7   the inability of staff to express feelings of fear and anxiety may be generated by male attitudes of perceived weakness

KEY POINTS

By now the reader will be aware that:

- ☐   Ethnic minority personnel are under-represented in management positions.
- ☐   Racial violence is under-reported.
- ☐   Institutionalised racism is prevalent within many social care settings.
- ☐   Institutional racism requires proactive approaches if it is to be eradicated.
- ☐   Racial violence is often considered less important than other forms of violence.
- ☐   Much can be done to reduce racism in social care.
- ☐   A macho workplace culture reduces the likelihood of violence being reported and therefore managed appropriately.
- ☐   Male attitudes can contribute to a maintenance of violence.
- ☐   Women are under-represented in senior management positions.
- ☐   Women form the majority of workers within social care.
- ☐   It is a sign of strength to be aware of and able to express fear and anxiety.
- ☐   Gender issues can play their part in the management of aggression.

REFERENCES

1 *The Stephen Lawrence Inquiry*. Report of an inquiry by Sir William Macpherson of Cluny. February 1999. The Stationery Office.

2 Smith, P. K. (1994) 'Social development', in A. M. Coleman (ed.) *Companion Encyclopaedia of Psychology*. Volume 2. Routledge, p. 731.

3 Barton, M. (2nd edn, 1997) *Ethnic and Racial Consciousness*. Longman.

4 Barker, M. (1981) *The New Racism: Conservatives and the Ideology of the Tribe*. Junction Books.

5 'The general duty to promote racial equality. Guidance for public authorities on their obligations under the Race Relations (Amendment) Act 2000' (2001). Pamphlet commissioned by the CRE. Available as a free PDF file from: www.cre.gov.uk/

6 Thompson, A. 'What happened to equality?' *Community Care*. 20–26 July 2000. An article which discusses the reasons why so few managers within social care are people from ethnic minorities.

7 See 6 above.

8 Economic and Social Research Council (1998) *Taking Stock*. ESRC Violence Research Programme. Brunel University, Uxbridge, Middlesex UB8 3PH.

9 Balloch, S., McLean, J. and Fisher, M. (eds) (1999) *Social Services: Working under Pressure*. Policy Press.

10 White, C. 'Keeping violence in mind.' *Community Care*. 28 Oct.–3 Nov. 1999.

KEY READING

Braham, P., Rattansi, A. and Skellington, R. (eds) (1992) *Racism and Anti-racism: Inequalities, Opportunities and Policies*. Sage.

Hilton, A. and Roberts, J. 'Danger men at work.' *Community Care*. 22–28 April 1999.
Huber, N. 'Black social workers still looking up at a glass ceiling.' *Community Care*. 14–20 Oct. 1999.
Webb, R. and Tossell, D. (1991) *Social Issues for Carers. A Community Care Perspective*. Edward Arnold.

Useful websites for information about ethnic issues:
www.blink.org.uk
www.kingsfund.org.uk

The Commission for Racial Equality operates from: 10–12 Allington Street, London SW1E 5EH (Tel: 0207 828 7022). They will also have the number of your local Racial Equality Council.

CHAPTER 8

THE CONSEQUENCES OF AGGRESSION

In this chapter I want to consider some of the elements occurring after a violent incident. In particular, by making use of ABC charting, a learning tool available to us all, I want to examine some of the consequences experienced after violence, in order to help the reader learn from past events.

This chapter will examine the consequences pertinent to:

- you
- the perpetrator
- other staff
- other service users

OBJECTIVES

By the end of the chapter you should be aware of:

- The psychological impacts of aggression upon the victim.

- Some ways in which perpetrators are responded to.

- Arguments for and against police involvement.

- Impacts of violence upon a work team.

- Effects of violence upon those not central to the incident yet still influenced by it.

I have included examples of ABC charting[1] to identify and learn from situations. I have also included a debriefing model which has been used successfully, helping many people who have experienced violence to adjust to the trauma and stress generated.

ABC CHARTING AND THE CONSEQUENCES OF VIOLENCE

An ABC chart can be an invaluable method for identifying and learning from elements occurring within a violent incident. The elements covered by the chart are shown in Figure 8.1.

1 ANTECEDENTS (a) history (b) immediate	2 BEHAVIOUR and 3 WAY MANAGED	4 CONSEQUENCES (a) to you (b) to the perpetrator (c) to other staff (d) to other service users
1 (a) Elements covered should include all those facts you have identified that are pertinent to the situation (see Chapter 3). 1 (b) Identify any possible triggers that may have sparked a reaction. Consider the events occurring immediately prior to the event, especially those occurring up to one hour beforehand (see Chapter 2).	2 Describe specifically the actual behaviour and/or words used (see Chapter 1). 3 Give a clear description of what was said and/or done to manage the behaviour at that time (see Chapter 5).	4 (a) Identify any personal impacts that are directly related to this event, both emotional or practical. 4 (b) Consider what happened to the perpetrator? Did he/she have the behaviour rewarded or sanctioned? How? 4 (c) Sometimes incidents can unite or split a work team. Individuals and/or performance may be criticised or praised. What impact did the situation have on your team functioning? 4 (d) Identify how other service users may have been affected.

Figure 8.1 ABC chart

ACTIVITY 8.1

With two colleagues:

- Making use of the above chart, each person in turn describe a situation where they faced aggression.

- One participant tells their story, another asks questions helping to elicit information and the third person makes notes. Take at least fifteen minutes for each situation.

- Finally identify: what were the learning points from completing the ABC chart?

Elements 1 to 3 have already been considered within this workbook. Those identified under 4 (Consequences) above are the elements I intend to now cover. They are the consequences:

- TO YOU
- TO THE PERPETRATOR
- TO THE STAFF TEAM
- TO OTHER SERVICE USERS

CONSEQUENCES TO YOU

The personal aftermath of violence

You are important. You are the most important component your agency is ever likely to have and looking after you is crucial. Because the effects of violence can be long-lasting and debilitating it is important to ensure that the emotional impacts generated by the incident are addressed appropriately. In order to address these impacts we need first to identify them.

The psychological impacts of violence include:

- PERFORMANCE GUILT
- RECONSTRUCTION ANXIETY
- IRRITABILITY
- FOCUSED RESENTMENT OR ANGER
- LOSS OF MOTIVATION

Performance guilt is the process whereby we assume responsibility for causing the incident even when this is simply not the case. There are a number of reasons why we do this:

1   we do not to want to blame the individual who has damaged us because of their circumstances

2   we are the professional and believe that we should know how to prevent situations
3   we blame ourselves as a means of attempting to explain the situation in terms
      that will give us some control over future events

Performance guilt can be identified as self-doubt, and typical thoughts or expressions
include: 'if only I'd not said that . . . if only I'd not done that . . . if only I'd not gone
into that room' or 'it wouldn't have happened if I hadn't . . .'

Performance guilt can be erosive and can stop us from believing in our skills and
abilities. The advice I give is: by all means examine your performance and if you want
to change it in future then do so, but stop blaming yourself, especially if you treated the
person with dignity and respect. Do not give violence an excuse; instead examine the
situation and identify ways that may prevent it from occurring in the future, if possible.

Reconstruction anxiety is the unbidden replaying of the event in the mind. This
could happen in sleep where the event repeats in dreams, or while awake where it occurs
as a 'flashback' often triggered by an association with the event such as a sight, sound
or smell. This is not uncommon. You may, for example, be walking down a street when
you see someone who reminds you of your assailant and suddenly you begin to re-
experience some of the emotions and physiological changes that occurred at the time
of the incident.

Reconstruction anxiety is a natural process allowing the mind and body to readjust
to the trauma experienced. For many of us this trauma includes emotional changes
of shock, horror, embarrassment, rejection, denial, and even attraction and excitement.
Simultaneously physiological changes include rapid breathing, heart racing, increased
blood pressure, trembling, coloration changes, etc. All of these can occur almost
instantaneously during the incident. The mind and body need time to readjust to these
changes and reconstruction anxiety is a part of that process. If the reconstructions do
not abate over time it may become necessary to do something. Talking can help; writing
the event down, actively recalling the event when you are feeling calm and in control,
and drawing are all processes which have worked for others. Sometimes counselling or
some other more professional therapeutic help may be required.

Irritability – we feel irritable with:

- ourselves because we think we should have handled the situation better
- our colleagues because where were they when they were needed?
- our manager because he/she should have known it was going to happen and should
  have prevented it
- our loved ones because they do not realise the awful day we have just experienced

Try to manage the irritability generated at the time by taking a break and talking to
colleagues. Alternatively go somewhere in private and shout at the universe, cry or do
something active to get rid of it. If you get home in a bit of a state, forewarn your loved
ones before snapping, shouting or provoking that row which is really nothing to do with
them. When you arrive home in an irritable state, say to your partner 'I need some
time', and go and luxuriate in a bath or clean the car to allow the irritability to dissipate.
If you do take it out on a loved one, apologise afterwards.

Focused resentment or anger can be harder to deal with as it is usually more deeply
rooted than the surface irritability. The resentment and anger felt are not necessarily
directed towards the person who damaged us; instead they may surface elsewhere.

Within the reserved British culture many of us find it hard to acknowledge that we are angry and harder still to express it constructively. There are many reasons for this:

- we often associate anger with violence
- we are taught that it is somehow wrong to express this emotion, that we must keep a lid on it for fear that it will damage or destroy
- some of us tend to think that anger is a flaw or weakness in our make-up
- it is perceived as something for service users and not something found within us

Anger is a valid emotion and can move mountains if it is used constructively. However, because of the inability to acknowledge or express it constructively, anger is frequently expressed destructively. Often the emotion leaks out suddenly, exploding disproportionately on to another who may well have inadvertently triggered the reaction by an insignificant act or omission.

Sometimes the suppressed anger can be internalised, appearing then in the physical form of headaches or migraine, a rise in blood pressure, hair loss, skin disorder, etc. It may produce sleeping or eating disorders. It may influence and distort perception and can bring about depression, or changes in thought pattern, and even lead to the desire for, or act of, revenge, thereby turning the victim into aggressor.

Focused resentment or anger can be managed by:

(a) Constructively letting the anger go. Actively plan to do something constructive the next time you are angry, to replace any destructive acts (see Chapter 9).

(b) Forgiveness. This is a form of internal forgiveness where we identify who created this feeling, what they did to generate this feeling, what impact their action(s) had upon us, and what changes this action generated in our lives. We then need to make a statement such as 'and it was not fair' or 'it should not have happened'. Finally we need to then say to ourselves, preferably out loud, 'However I now forgive [name] for it.' Then we mean it.

(c) Addressing the emotion with the person concerned. Where appropriate and usually following on from (a) or (b), go to the person involved and say: '*I feel angry, can I talk to you about it?*' Tell of the behaviour that created this feeling within you and offer an alternative way in which the person could have behaved differently. (Note – this will not always work and it is necessary to make an assessment of the person you are to approach, as some people will gain a sense of satisfaction from knowing that they have generated this feeling within you, and others can consider the discussion of emotion as a sign of weakness.)

ACTIVITY 8.2

In a group or individually:

Think about how you manage your anger and make a list of those things you do when you are in an angry state.

Next, with a colleague identify how the negative expressions of this emotion, which may be damaging you, your image or another person, can be turned into a positive action.

Loss of motivation is commonly experienced either following an accumulation of what may be thought of as minor incidents or after a major event. It is the gradual withdrawal from situations that previously we felt able to deal with, and can be identified in such phrases as: '*I'm not going to ask those challenging questions I previously asked. . . . I've been damaged before. . . . Let someone else do it for a change. . . . Let them know what it feels like.*' This then develops into negativity, cynicism and hostile feelings.

In order to counter loss of motivation I ask the individual to concentrate upon her/his successes and to praise those successes appropriately. This becomes important because we are not praised enough for our achievements and many of us tend not to praise ourselves at all, often believing that self-praise is sycophantic. Yet we will regularly criticise our own performance. This imbalance needs addressing as it is a root cause for loss of motivation. On a day-to-day basis, therefore, identify four things that you have done successfully, focus upon these things and give yourself praise for these achievements.

The needs of the person subjected to violence

Following an aggressive incident, those involved may experience a combination of the above impacts. Many will need no more than a sympathetic colleague or friend providing understanding and solace, helping to identify and work through the emotions experienced. Some of us may need more.

ACTIVITY 8.3

In a group identify:

1 What should be done for a colleague who has experienced violence at work:

   (a) if the incident has only just occurred?
   (b) if the colleague has been at home 'off sick' for two weeks?

2 What would you want to happen if this were you?

The points listed below have often been found useful:

- access to others who have experienced violence and adjusted
- someone to take immediate control of the situation
- immediate decisions taken by another
- help to overcome feelings of loss of security, guilt and self-blame
- time to readjust
- time and opportunity to discuss the incident
- exploration of the way forward
- a clear choice of future contact with the aggressor
- to be positively reacted to by colleagues
- information about insurance, compensation, legal and other rights
- someone to turn to
- not to be interrogated

Emotional debriefing model

Many working units offer the opportunity of debriefing to staff who have been subjected to violence. Debriefing need not be left solely to the confines of a professional counsellor; it can be provided by suitable personnel within the workplace. However, the person completing the debriefing requires guidance, and the following model is provided for this purpose.

Although it is difficult to estimate the number and length of debriefing sessions required, my advice is to offer up to four one-hour sessions, with the first session allowing for a discussion of the whole event and the remaining three sessions making use of the following model. Use the model in a linear form, from left to right, asking the person to talk through their experience (see Figure 8.2).

	WHAT SPECIFIC FACTS DO YOU REMEMBER?	HOW WERE YOU FEELING?	WHAT WERE YOU SPECIFICALLY PHYSICALLY DOING TO EXPRESS THOSE FEELINGS?
BEFORE THE INCIDENT			
WHILE THE INCIDENT WAS OCCURRING			
IMMEDIATELY FOLLOWING THE INCIDENT			
NOW WITH HINDSIGHT			

Figure 8.2 Emotional debriefing model

Ripple effects[2]

Anyone who has experienced a violent incident will know that, besides the above, there are many other more subtle impacts and changes occurring which are related to the incident yet which appear so insignificant as to be not worth considering. The effects could become part of a 'hardening-up' process, or they could involve a change in attitudes, a readjustment of priorities or even a change in the way others function around us.

It is like the effect of throwing a stone into a still pond – first there is the impact, and once this is ended the ripples radiate outwards changing the appearance of the pond as they do so. As these ripple effects often occur following violence, influencing individuals and working units, they should not be ignored.

Typical ripple effect

Incident occurs and care worker affected ~~~ worker goes home, talks to partner ~~~ partner becomes angry, insists worker is not to return to work ~~~ care worker and partner argue ~~~ care worker decides not to tell partner of any future incidents, thereby severing possible support system.

ACTIVITY 8.4

Working in a small group with colleagues:

1 Identify a situation where aggression took place within your working unit.

2 Make a list of who was involved and identify with those colleagues the ripple effects experienced.

CONSEQUENCES TO THE PERPETRATOR

The following are examples of ABC charts completed by course participants using the procedure outlined in Activity 8.1. The charts are completed in note form and the consequences to the perpetrator have been highlighted.

1 ANTECEDENTS (a) history (b) immediate	2 BEHAVIOUR and 3 WAY MANAGED	4 CONSEQUENCES (a) to you **(b) to perpetrator** (c) to other staff (d) to other service users
Case 1 1(a) 14-year-old child with history of absconding from placements. Unsettled history – spending time with	2 Child angry and reluctant to get into car with social work assistant. Cajoled into it. On way asked if she could smoke. Opened	4(a) Devastated. It was my first week in social care – off sick for three weeks. Medical check-up. Inquiry held because

different family members when parents rowed. Parents drug abusers. Mother often hit by partner. Poor school attendance. Becoming involved in drug scene. Violent towards teachers. Moved out of county to sever drug links.

1(b) On second day in placement needed some clothes. Truculent all morning. Refused breakfast. Did not want to go shopping.

window and she kicked and headbutted me and ran off.

3 Chased her and grabbed her wrist. She turned and slapped me in the face. Let her go.
Told afterwards that I was silly for chasing her.

of bruising to child's wrist. Told not to hold children who are absconding in future. Told to read policy document. Felt complete failure.

4(b) Girl returned that night and was praised for returning. No action taken over assault.

4(c) Other staff mostly supportive said 'You'll learn.'

4(d) Girl became like a hero to some. Group formed who became bullies. Eventually needed to be split up.

Case 2
1(a) Both are chronic alcoholics – dry for over six months. He has history of mental health problems. Long-standing relationship. Little money. Living in high-rise council block. Ongoing dispute with one set of neighbours. Good relationship with others.

1(b) Phone call previous day saying he had discovered her to be involved with another man.

2 On home visit it became clear that he had been drinking that day. Refused to let me leave. Pushed me into bedroom where she was sleeping it off. Threatened me with a kitchen knife.

3 Sat on bed and when he came towards me rushed out past him.

4(a) Shaking, sweating. Deflated and feeling a failure. Nightmares even now two years later.

4(b) Clients now told will only be seen in office.

4(c) Blamed by other staff members for not 'reading' the situation better beforehand.

4(d) Female client is left alone with him – no checks – is told she will only be seen in office – she has not made contact.

Case 3

1(a) No history available –
client unknown.

1(b) Duty system started at 9.
Man immediately
entered building and
demanded to see social
worker. Duty social
worker still not arrived.
Receptionist told man
he would have to wait.
Man appeared confused
and inarticulate? mental
health or maybe not
English. Living in bail
hostel. Wanted help in
getting new
accommodation.

2 While waiting began to
toss magazines on to floor.
Then started to kick table
while sitting – his leg
rocking into table leg.
Shouted at receptionist
that he needed to see a
social worker. Began
swearing and banging
counter.

3 Female social worker
arrived through front
door, walked up to man
and told him the police
would be called if he
did not leave. Man left
smashing door window
with his fist.

4(a) Receptionist in tears.
Social worker shaken.
Both afraid to leave
building at lunchtime.
Receptionist asked for
and given new job away
from reception.

**4(b) Service user was not
seen.**

4(c) Lot of anger and
accusations. Social worker
blamed for being late.
Managers blamed for
allowing duty system to
operate without duty
officer.

4(d) Less time for other
clients as duty system now
reduced to 10 to 4 –
previously 9 till 5.

Case 4

1(a) History of children
being in care. Children
neglected and on
register. Previous
violence involving
couple and directed
towards children.
Unemployed. Debt
problems. Working
with couple but they
are resentful because of
my colour and have
asked for a white
worker.

1(b) Message from
neighbours that children
left alone all night.
Big fight between couple.

2 Arrived and found him
alone. Reluctant to let me
in initially. Said the
children were in the
bedroom. Went in but
they were not. He
followed and closed the
door behind him. Started
to make sexual remarks
and began to touch my
arm and shoulder.

3 Firm boundaries. Told him
not to talk to me like that
and not to touch me
again. Then left.

4(a) Felt dirty, oppressed,
threatened. Ambiguous
feelings of anxiety for
children and desire
not to visit again.

**4(b) Power. He had the
ability to do this sort of
thing and get away
with it.**

4(c) Shared experiences
and consoled each other.
Was given the support
required to enable me to
return and make sure
children were OK.

4(d) Less time available to
other service users
because of time-
consuming demands
to ensure children's
safety.

Case 5		
1(a) Person known for these sorts of comments. 1(b) Working together in residential unit for people with learning difficulties.	2 Colleague said 'You probably don't know it but in this country it's polite to ask before doing something.' 3 Challenged her racist assumption that I am not from this country. Took it up with the manager who said it was just the way she was and not to let it worry me.	4(a) Felt angry – unable to carry on as if nothing had happened. **4(b) Became empowered by the various incidents and the way they were not managed by the manager.** 4(c) Caused division in staff team – resentment. 4(d) Lack of motivation towards my clients.

In the above cases it becomes obvious that the consequences experienced by the individual worker are far greater than those borne by the perpetrator of the act of violence. In brief, these are:

	TO STAFF MEMBER	TO PERPETRATOR
Case 1	Devastated. It was my first week in social care – off sick for three weeks. Medical check-up. Inquiry held because of bruising to child's wrist. Told not to hold children who are absconding in future. Told to read policy document. Felt complete failure.	Girl returned that night and was praised for returning. No action taken over assault.
Case 2	Shaking, sweating. Deflated and feeling a failure. Nightmares even now two years later.	Clients now told will only be seen in office.
Case 3	Receptionist in tears. Social worker shaken. Both afraid to leave building at lunchtime. Receptionist asked for and given new job away from reception.	Service user was not seen.
Case 4	Felt dirty, oppressed, threatened. Ambiguous feelings of anxiety for children and desire not to visit again.	Power. He had the ability to do this sort of thing and get away with it.
Case 5	Felt angry – unable to carry on as if nothing had happened.	Became empowered by the various incidents and the way they were not managed by the manager.

ACTIVITY 8.5

Individually, or in a group, identify:

What should be the consequences of the perpetrator's actions in the above cases?

Police involvement

With the above situations there is no reference to police involvement being a consequence of the perpetrator's actions – even in those situations where an assault took place, the police were not involved. I find this disturbing, especially when considering the comparison between the apparent lack of responsibility for the behaviour experienced by the perpetrators and the impact felt by the workers. What is equally disturbing is the acceptance of violence perpetrated upon others within our presence which may go unreported.

CASE STUDY

You have been asked to call in to see Susan (19 years) on your way home, in order to give her some information about her child's operation. Susan has been well known to your agency for some time and you have seen her on numerous occasions in your building. You knock at the door which is soon opened by Susan who appears very rushed.

Before you can say anything she invites you in, turns and walks down the hallway leading into the lounge. You follow after closing the door behind you and are now standing in the door frame which leads into the lounge. On the opposite side of the room to you is the door leading to the kitchen. Sprawled on the settee you see a man (aged 19/20 years) whom you do not know watching TV.

Susan picks up a mug of tea from the small table and the man sits up as she puts the mug by his feet, accidentally spilling some. 'You stupid cow', he says as he slaps her hard across the face.

Susan rushes out of the room crying and holding her cheek. She has run into the kitchen – the room directly opposite to where you are standing. The man throws you a look which says, 'And what's it to you?' He then leans back on the settee and resumes his viewing.

ACTIVITY 8.6

In a mixed-gender group identify:

1 What would you do next and why?

2 Are there any gender differences in the way this situation would be handled?

3 Would you report this incident to the police?

Arguments often given for not reporting such situations to the police include:

- the police will treat it as a 'domestic' and will not want to become involved
- the victim must give her consent for the worker to report it
- it would destroy the trust between the service user and the worker
- it is the responsibility of the victim to report the matter

Reasons for reporting include:

- you have witnessed an assault
- domestic violence is a criminal offence
- the police now regard any act of domestic violence as a serious matter
- domestic violence units have been established to deal sensitively with all reported incidents
- victims of domestic violence are repeatedly assaulted before seeking help
- failure to report makes you an accessory after the fact
- you are in an official capacity and have therefore a greater responsibility to report such situations

From my experience I have found the involvement of the police uncommon in social care, in particular police involvement within residential and day-care units where violence occurs.

CASE STUDY

Helen (22 years) is a person with severe learning difficulties living in a residential unit which prides itself on managing challenging behaviours. Earlier today she was to have gone out with her key worker but unfortunately this had to be cancelled. She was not told why. Helen had spent the morning watching TV in the main lounge. Two of the other residents Judith (19 years) and Simon (20 years) had been larking about and had been told off once already by one of the care staff for disturbing Helen.

Judith decided that she wanted to sit where Helen was sitting and slid from the arm of the chair, squeezing into the small space left by Helen. The two began to push at each other. Unfortunately, Helen's fingernail caught Judith in the face and Judith erupted with a screech. Simon rushed over and began pulling at Helen's hair and, although resisting, she was gradually lifted by her hair from the seat and pulled to one side of the chair. It was at this point that the care officer who had come in to see what was happening shouted 'Stop that' at Simon. Helen fell to the floor, while Simon still held a handful of her hair. Judith sat back tutting loudly.

ACTIVITY 8.7

Consider individually, or in a group discuss:

If you were the care officer would you notify the police of this incident of assault? Give your reasons.

The arguments for not involving the police within residential and day-care units include:

- service user lacks capacity to bring an action
- service user lacks credibility to bring an action
- negative reactions from the police who consider such actions a normal occurrence within care establishments
- police do not want to get involved with our service users
- it will jeopardise the trust and relationship between worker and service users
- it is a disruption to other service users
- it creates a drama and rewards bad behaviour as the police pick the offender up and take them for a nice drive in a police car
- unreliable witnesses to the incident mean nothing will be done
- it is bad publicity for the working unit
- pressure of work
- it should be dealt with internally
- guilt by staff who feel they should manage it
- admission of failure

The arguments in favour of police involvement include:

- service users have the same rights as everyone else
- the perpetrator has broken the law and police involvement reinforces this
- it protects other service users
- it gives a clear message that such behaviour is unacceptable
- it is empowering to the victim
- police presence can stop escalation
- information gathered by the police may identify dangerous individuals
- it helps to build up a body of evidence
- it protects staff from criticism
- it demystifies the roles of care staff and police and builds relationships.
- the unit has a responsibility to protect service users
- the perpetrator needs to be held accountable
- Criminal Injuries Compensation will not be payable unless notification is made

CONSEQUENCES TO THE STAFF TEAM

Violence can affect the staff team in a variety of ways. In some instances the incident may serve to unite the team by:

- focusing the team upon ensuring the non-recurrence of future incidents
- allowing individuals to focus upon the needs of the damaged colleague(s)
- identifying the positive elements in the work
- encouraging open communication
- identifying working practices and shoring-up any weak areas
- identifying constructive criticism and enabling appropriate feedback
- reawakening personal safety issues

ACTIVITY 8.8

In a work-team where violence has been experienced by one or more staff, discuss:

What were the impacts of the violent incident upon the team and its functioning?

Frequently there can be adverse reactions by individuals which may highlight chinks in what was previously considered smooth team functioning. Some examples of this may be perceived in the ABC cases already identified:

Case 1: *Other staff mostly supportive said 'You'll learn.'* Although the term 'supportive' is used by the care worker involved, the additional 'You'll learn' appears to suggest the culture of inevitability, indicating that future situations will occur, rather than a genuine desire to ensure non-recurrence.

Case 2: *Blamed by other staff members for not 'reading' the situation better beforehand.* This reaction clearly identifies the need for team building with opportunities for constructive and non-critical forms of feedback. Otherwise the resentment and anger generated by this situation will cause the team involved to split and lead to demotivated and non-committed staff.

Case 3: *Lot of anger and accusations. Social worker blamed for being late. Managers blamed for allowing duty system to operate without duty officer.* Here the situation is even worse than above. The team(s) involved will need the opportunity to openly vent their anger in a safe environment before being able to move on. Open communication about expectations, roles and responsibilities is always desirable before any incident. Indeed it is the role of the manager and the responsibility of all workers to create an atmosphere where all staff can talk openly about violence or its possibility.

Case 4: *Shared experiences and consoled each other. Was given the support required to enable me to return and make sure children were OK.* Here the worker returned to a dangerous situation because of her anxiety for the safety of the children, and the reason for this appears to be directly related to the 'support' provided by the team. This team can be at risk of over-support, whereby individual staff actively place themselves in a risky situation for fear of letting the team down. An alternative supportive approach is for another colleague to accompany the worker, or for the team to discuss the possibility of the worker returning accompanied by the police.

Case 5: *Caused division in staff team – resentment.* Once again the individuals making up this team require the opportunity to openly discuss the team processes. This should occur at team meetings, during individual supervision, or in three-way or other meetings involving an outside enabler experienced in team communication skills.

With all the above cases there is an argument for helping staff to communicate effectively. One approach that has often been found helpful is to make use of the elements contained within constructive feedback.

Constructive feedback (see also 'Assertiveness', Chapter 5, p. 88):

- is the process whereby information is provided to an individual or group of workers about performance, in a manner which the person(s) perceives as helpful and which will enable the person(s) concerned to change future performance

- has been found to be most helpful when invited and when agreed by all concerned

- is most productive when given within three days of the event concerned

- is given by one individual who uses 'I' terminology

- focuses upon performance and/or behaviour

- seeks clarification, e.g. 'David do you remember yesterday when you lifted Susan?'

- links performance and impact, e.g. 'David, when you lifted Susan like [description] it made me feel very uncomfortable . . .'

- provides an alternative way to achieve what the previous performance achieved '. . . and in future I would like you to . . . [describe alternative]'

- provides a reason 'I would like you to . . . [describe alternative] . . . because it could be misconstrued . . .'

- is concerned for the person who is receiving the information '. . . and I know that's not the case and I wouldn't want anyone to think that about you'

- asks for feedback, e.g. 'Are you OK with that?'

CONSEQUENCES TO OTHER SERVICE USERS

Additionally, the effects of violence can be experienced by other individuals, some of whom may not have been involved in the event.

CASE STUDY

Mrs Shields, known as Daisy, had been a resident in Deenhaven for nearly six years and enjoyed her daily routine of washing (now needing some assistance), breakfast, the morning in the day lounge, or on a good day some of it spent in the garden, and then an activity in the afternoon after lunch. Occasionally she dozed through the early evening until tea, watched some television and then went to bed. She knew most of the other residents and was a real help settling in new people. She was 84 when the incident occurred.

For some months now there had been an influx of new residents, with a number being transferred from other homes which had closed because of a lack of finance. She was a little confused with so many new faces but put a good face on it herself and remained 'chirpy' – a word used by one of her favourite care staff to describe her. The day lounge was noisier now than she liked, but then she told herself it took new people some time to settle in. It was a bright Tuesday in late September, her favourite month, the month she had married, though no one seemed to know that now save herself. A couple of residents had been rowing earlier in the day, which had unsettled many of the others, and Daisy decided she would prefer to be in the garden rather than the day lounge. Unfortunately there were not enough staff on and so the garden was out of bounds and the door locked. She edged herself around with her walking frame and began making her way back towards the lounge, when bedlam broke loose. The two who had been arguing were now shouting angrily and the noise suggested objects were being thrown. Bert Makin came from the lounge and was panting in the doorway as two care staff rushed past him to deal with the two who were creating the havoc. Suddenly the fire alarm went off. Daisy was stunned. Her peaceful day shattered. She made her way slowly back to her room suddenly feeling very alone and very afraid. Her good mood gone she closed the bedroom door and knew that everything was changed.

ACTIVITY 8.9

In a group discuss:

1 When violence occurs within a residential or day-care unit, besides dealing with the immediate situation, what else is required?

2 What should be done for Daisy?

3 What happens within your unit for those not directly involved?

In the above case study it is obvious that this incident impacted upon another resident and that she (Daisy) would be needing staff involvement to help her readjust, or simply someone to talk to.

In many situations of violence others besides those directly involved are often affected. Other service users may require:

- acknowledgement that the situation occurred
- the opportunity to discuss fears generated by the event
- formal debriefing
- time to readjust
- the chance to regain normality as soon as possible
- reassurance that the situation will not be repeated
- information about the victim and the aggressor, e.g. when will they return?

KEY POINTS

This chapter has considered the consequences of violence, and by now you should be aware of how:

☐   To complete an ABC chart following an aggressive incident.

☐   A violent incident can have an impact upon the victim(s), perpetrator(s), team functioning and other service users.

☐   Psychological impacts can be managed.

☐   Emotional debriefing can help in this process.

☐   Ripple effects may also need addressing.

☐   The responsibility held by the perpetrator for his/her behaviour is often overlooked.

☐   Police involvement can be a valuable element.

☐   Team cohesiveness may be affected by violence.

☐   Constructive feedback can help to open up communication within teams.

☐   Other service users can be affected and may require help in readjusting.

ABC charting can help clarify the processes involved when violent incidents occur. It can also provide useful clues for preventing, avoiding or managing future incidents.

REFERENCES

1   Sheldon, B. (1995) *Cognitive-behavioural Therapy: Research, Practice and Philosophy.* Routledge.
2   Lawrence, C. (ed.) (1993) *The Security Journal.* Perpetuity Press. Describes research carried out at the University of Leicester into the ripple effects of violence upon a team.

KEY READING

Braithwaite, R. 'Coming to terms with the effects of violence.' *Social Work Today.* 20 Oct. 1988.

Hunter, M. 'How violence strikes.' *Community Care.* 29 July–4 Aug. 1999. Two workers who have been subjected to violence report on their feelings.

Hunter, M. 'Supporting front line staff.' *Community Care.* 5–11 Aug. 1999. Identifies one council's policies on violence to staff.

Hunter, M.'Time to get a grip.' *Community Care.* 19–25 Aug. 1999. Considers the psychological effects of violence upon a team.

CHAPTER 9

ALTERNATIVES TO AGGRESSION

In this chapter I want to consider some of the alternative ways to express aggression. The chapter will identify some strategies that allow service users to successfully express anger and frustration other than in the form of aggression.

It becomes important to consider alternative ways of expressing these emotions for two reasons:

1   Many individuals have no alternatives, no other ways of expressing anger, simply because of limited education in this field.
2   There is nothing wrong with anger or indeed with being frustrated. There is a lot wrong, however, when either of these emotions is expressed negatively as aggression which damages ourselves or others.

Furthermore, providing alternative ways to express anger and frustration is fundamental in a system where we are saying to the service user 'stop this aggressive behaviour'. If we fail to provide alternative ways to express these valid emotions, we will be guilty of further disadvantaging service users and I believe we will ultimately fail to stop the rise of aggression within society.

OBJECTIVES

By the end of the chapter the reader will be aware of some:

▪   Individual strategies.

▪   Group initiatives.

These will help to reduce aggression by replacing it with alternative approaches.

There are a number of alternatives available to anyone which can help replace the need to be aggressive. These alternatives can be placed under the following headings:

- individual responses
- group work

INDIVIDUAL RESPONSES AVAILABLE TO SERVICE USERS

Befriending

I am frequently amazed at the intuition of many care workers who, often without training, offer their service user the opportunity to change their aggressive behaviour. This was re-emphasised only recently when, during a training session for care staff, I asked the participants to identify the alternatives to aggression they offered to their clients. One domiciliary care officer replied 'knitting' and, although a couple of her colleagues laughed, I asked her to explain.

EDITH'S STORY

Well, I was visiting this old woman. She was about 80 and had been on her own since her husband died for about four years. All the home helps who knew them liked them a lot, but after he died she became very morose and a bit withdrawn. Anyway, she stopped the [domiciliary care] service and we hadn't heard from her for a couple of years when she was re-referred by the GP. So I was asked to go in. I was shocked at the change. Not only in her appearance – she was thin and tended not to wash or change her clothes, things like that – but it was in her mood. She was really angry. She used to shout and throw things when she could get them at anyone in the house. It was getting to the point that we were thinking of stopping the service because, although she hadn't hurt anyone, some of the staff were really afraid of her. Anyway, I said to her one day 'Do you knit?' She could see well enough and she didn't have arthritis or anything like that so I thought I would give it a go, and after a bit of a protest from her I said 'Look May. I think you're lonely and you won't go out to a day centre or anything, so I'll come here and teach you to knit if you like. It's up to you. What do you think?'

Anyway she didn't say anything then but she must have thought about it because the next time I went she said 'Yes'. So I started to call around. Twice a week was all I could manage but that seemed to do it. I taught her how to knit and had chats with her while we were doing it and she just stopped shouting and throwing things at people.

ACTIVITY 9.1

As an individual identify, or in a group discuss:

What alternatives do you offer to your service users to allow them to express their anger and/or frustration?

In the above example Edith chose to befriend May, which I applaud because she:

- provided company
- gave her client the chance to talk
- taught her client new skills
- provided her client with a feeling of self-worth

I am, however, concerned that an individual approach like this may place the provider in a potentially dangerous and unmonitored situation. I am also concerned that should Edith have been the subject of aggression she would not have been covered by her agency's insurance.

Befriending schemes can be extremely valuable, yet so often they rely upon the goodwill of volunteers and are not necessarily an integral part of formal social care. This could place many of the volunteers engaged within the process at risk.

Do you have a befriending scheme in your area? What is the referral process?

Empowerment

Empowerment is the process whereby the service user is enabled to achieve or attempt to achieve their goals with the support, but without the formal intervention, of a care worker. This may involve giving the service user information – for example, about the complaints procedure – and the appropriate help to use this effectively. Alternatively, providing the service user with useful contacts – whether that be appropriate pressure groups or simply the names of local councillors who may be able to assist – is equally valid. It may involve enabling the service user to actively lobby or demonstrate. True empowerment, however, is often precluded by the agency policy which formally or informally frowns upon the voicing of any dissatisfaction; and real empowerment may come from advocacy systems.

Advocacy systems

Over the last 20 years or so, advocacy services for looked after children have developed in a largely ad hoc way. Since the 1989 Children Act a number of councils have appointed their own children's rights officers or have commissioned advocacy services for looked after children. This is in addition to Schedule 2 of the Children Act to appoint an independent visitor in respect of any looked after child who is not being regularly visited when they believe it would be in the best interest of the child. However the role of the independent visitor does not amount to being an advocate.

Lost in Care[1] provides many examples of children who attempted to complain about an unhappy situation but whose voices were not heard.[2]

ACTIVITY 9.2

In a group discuss:

1 What is an advocate?

2 What are the roles and responsibilities of an advocate?

3 Which service user may require an advocate?

Advocacy is about helping vulnerable people to make their wishes and needs known in order that they receive the appropriate aid or services which can improve the quality of their lives. Roles of the advocate include:

- Spokesperson: to vigorously represent the interests of the vulnerable person in situations where their rights are at risk of being compromised, neglected or abused.
- Enabler: helping the person to speak up for themselves.
- Information aide: finding information and useful contacts or groups who may act for the vulnerable person, and enabling the vulnerable person to make use of these contacts where appropriate.

In addition to advocacy systems for looked after children, *No Secrets*[3] gives local authorities the lead role in ensuring that vulnerable adults are provided with access to an independent advocate. This role comes into effect immediately and the necessary procedures must be in place by the end of October 2001.

Demonstrative approaches

Service users often look to staff for role models and examples. Unfortunately many of us are unable to provide positive models for constructively managing anger. This lack of productive anger management is frequently identified, especially in one training exercise where I ask participants to identify what they do when they are angry at home.

ACTIVITY 9.3

Individually list, or in a group brainstorm:

At home what do you do when you are really angry?

The following examples are typically provided:

- Shout and take it out on my partner
- Shout at the children
- Play loud music
- Have a drink

- Throw things
- Smoke
- Explode
- Play revenge fantasies over in my mind
- Speed up
- Grit my teeth
- Go quiet and sulk
- Drive more aggressively
- Spend a sleepless night
- Find it difficult to concentrate on anything else

Occasionally participants are able to identify some positive ways of dealing with their emotion, and these invariably include:

- Gardening
- Go for a run
- Housework
- Talk to a friend
- Tell those close to me that I am angry and ask them to give me a bit of space

My advice is clear – do something to LET THE ANGER GO. Unfortunately this is not easy, as many of us think that to let the anger leave us is to admit defeat. So we tend to keep hold of it only to have it manifest itself as a physical or psychological symptom (see Chapter 8). Once we can identify a mechanism for constructively letting go of the anger, we can then provide useful models for our service users.

CASE STUDY

Pat, who works in a small residential unit which accommodates six people with learning difficulties, explained how he learned to express his anger:

'Over the last few months I'd been becoming increasingly dissatisfied and disgruntled at work. I was short-tempered and snapping at the least little thing. Eventually things came to a head when one of the residents, Steve, lost his comb and accused me of failing to keep an eye on the other residents. It was the last straw and I knew that if I stayed around I would just blow. I had to walk out. I went into the garden and literally screamed. Steve had followed and I saw him stood in the kitchen. He'd turned white and I'm not surprised, but it was like a dam had burst in me. All the tension had gone. After a minute or two I walked back in and was able to sit with Steve to explain that I was really angry but that a lot of it was nothing to do with him at all.

Well, since that incident all of us in the house have been considering what we do with anger and what we can do to stop it exploding as aggression.'

ACTIVITY 9.4

In a group identify:

1 What are the disadvantages of such an approach?

2 What are the advantages?

How we let the anger go from us will vary from person to person. To find out what is best for you, identify what you do when you are angry and where necessary turn this into a positive technique. For example, if in temper you throw things, go to a car boot sale this weekend and purchase some old crockery; keep it in the garden and when you get to the point where you are about to blow go outside and throw that!

Other more tranquil ways of constructively letting the anger go may include meditation, writing, painting and talking.

ACTIVITY 9.5

With a group of service users discuss:

How does anger manifest itself within you/what do you do when you are angry?

Next, help your service users to identify a constructive method for expressing anger based upon their current negative mechanism.

Talking/counselling

Although the therapeutic value of talking has been repeatedly identified, the opportunity to talk is not readily available within many residential units, where the ratio of staff to residents may be as few as one to ten. Where time is spent on ensuring that the basics are achieved, sitting and talking are often frowned upon. Frequently, too, the type of education provided to the basic-grade residential worker fails to include counselling skills or reflective listening techniques, even in those situations where the worker is expected to become involved in personal care. Talking can help the aggressor to identify what may trigger an aggressive outburst, while also helping to identify other ways of responding.

Individual programme planning

Within one residential unit which caters for six people with learning difficulties, individual programme plans enable each of the residents to safely and appropriately express or manage their frustrations. Of the six residents, three have a physical disability and none of the six has the ability to vocalise their emotions. In the unit, the staffing ratio of three staff to six residents allows individual programme planning and its evaluation. The following is a brief outline of part of the individual programme planning used within the unit:

Service user:

(A)   has his own shed and uses this as personal space to get away from others when he feels frustrated.
(B)   tends to bang his head and kick at others when angry, so his bedroom has everything padded and he is able to retire there when necessary.
(C)   likes his hands massaged when he gets annoyed – it calms him and has reduced the really violent outbursts.
(D)   prefers to be quiet and will go into the garden or his own room.
(E)   needs to have someone to sit by him, without speaking – he just needs to know someone else is there.
(F)   likes reassurance that everything will be all right – he needs a friendly voice speaking in a calm manner.

Each of these methods is reviewed monthly and can be amended as required.

Time out

Time out involves enabling the person to leave a situation by going to a safe environment. In the above examples the opportunity of 'time out' was provided successfully for three of the residents.

Time out can be useful because it:

•   allows the emotion to dissipate
•   provides privacy for managing aggression – maybe as a controlled outburst or in the form of tears
•   reduces possible repercussions by minimising additional contacts with people who may otherwise become subjected to the aggression

Successful time out is never enforced.

Assertiveness

Assertive communication blends together the positive aspects of passivity and aggression. For the vast majority of us it is a learned method of communicating. Although initially it was felt to be most valuable for individuals who were more passive in their communication style, assertiveness has now been identified as being extremely productive in helping to replace aggression.

Teaching assertiveness skills to service users provides many with another means of achieving goals previously achieved via aggression. Assertiveness also encourages a positive self-image without denying the rights of others (see Chapter 5).

Direct work techniques

These techniques were first popularised in the 1980s when they were used to encourage children who had been abused to express their outrage and anger via controlled activities. These activities frequently included the use of sand, water and painting. Direction for the controlled expression of anger is provided by the worker who would, for example, ask the child to imagine their abuser is seated in an empty chair, and then with a bashing stick (rolled-up newspaper) hit the chair. Direct work techniques are used as a means of encouraging the child to express anger in a safe setting.

Use of such techniques requires knowledge and skill, and staff engaged in such a process should be trained in how to manage both the immediate situation and the potential outcomes.

How many staff within your working unit are trained in anger management skills?

Safe places

Safe places for expressing anger, such as Violence rooms, Music or Quiet rooms, are used within some establishments. Such rooms are used to contain the emotion and its expression, allowing the rest of the working unit to be effectively free of aggression.

GROUP WORK

Below are three examples of good practice where group work is specifically provided as a means of allowing individuals to express anger and/or frustration. There are many such group work schemes in operation nationwide and, although from my limited research in this area it appears that initial start-up funding for such projects may be relatively easy to obtain, ongoing funding to keep such valuable projects in operation is problematic.

ACTIVITY 9.6

In a group:

Make a list of the anger management group work schemes in your area.

What are the referral criteria for these units?

Group work example 1

In one centre in the London Borough of Sutton, young people aged between 10 and 17 years are given the opportunity of learning how to manage anger through the ritual and structure contained within judo. Robin Murly, the co-ordinator for the Judo Group, a part of the Family and Adolescent Support Team, explains: 'This is a specific anger management programme designed to allow young people to learn how to manage everyday situations without needing to resort to violence.'

The children, who may be at risk of coming into care or of foster breakdown because of their violence, attend a weekly session which uses judo as a focus while concentrating upon teaching the child social skills. The sessions are designed to provoke feelings within a controlled setting. Then, because the child has been taught the structured ritual of judo, when the feeling of anger is aroused, the ritual and structure allow the child to stop and think before acting. This enables the child to think through different approaches, different ways of achieving the same goal.

Furthermore, the entire process provides the child with:

- an awareness of anger
- identification of any triggers to which they react
- the opportunity to appraise the consequences of their actions

Additionally, the learning achieved is transferable into real-life situations. When confronted by situations that provoke anger in life, instead of immediately and instinctively responding, the child can call upon the different responses learned while attending the group.

The Judo Group has been running during term times for over five years, and has successfully dealt with between 40 and 50 children in this period. The groups are usually quite small, involving 6 to 8 participants with two instructors at any one time. Referral to the group is made through the London Borough of Sutton Family and Adolescent Support Team.

Group work example 2

Drawing cartoons of their own violent episodes and talking these through with other men convicted of domestic violence was one of the methods of self-examination used on a ten-week course managed by West Yorkshire Probation for offenders in 1996–7. The purpose of drawing the violent incident from beginning to end was to enable the men to face up to what they had done, which they previously had either denied or minimised. Once completed, each man had to describe to the group his own cartoon, identifying the causes, symptoms and triggers of the incident. Following the drawing and explanation, one incident was then chosen for use as a role-play session later in the course. Here the man selected for the role of the woman victim had to try to understand, probably for the first time, how it felt to be on the receiving end of such violence. Other men in the watching group were asked to empathise with the victim's role, which often created intense discomfort amongst the men.

In another session entitled 'My dad', participants were invited to consider their relationship with their father. In this session deep-seated and subconscious problems concerning the participant's desire or otherwise to emulate their father often surfaced.

Although it was felt that the course should be longer – but could not be, because of financial considerations – it appeared to be effective. Of the eight men who attended the pilot group, only two re-offended, and there has been continuously good feedback from participants.[4]

Group work example 3

'AWAKENS' (Abused Women And Kids Everyone Needs Support) is a project currently being run by Domestic Violence Services (Keighley). It is for women and children who have experienced domestic violence. Referrals come from Women's Aid, social services and the local Health Trusts of children whose behaviour is aggressive and disruptive at home and/or within school.

The project runs two groups simultaneously: one for children, the other for adults. Each group focuses upon the same issues, and the aim is to help the women and children to understand their experiences and to move on. Over a period of eight weeks, the weekly sessions – lasting one-and-a-half to two hours – concentrate on: defining domestic abuse; the feelings involved and provoked; safety and protection; power and stereotypes; conflict resolution; responsibility for the action; confidence and self-esteem building. Techniques used within the group sessions include: talking; story-telling and discussion; storyboard activities, where each child takes a turn to describe what is happening within a picture; speech bubbles, where children fill in a caption of what they think is going on in the mind of the cartoon image; question sheets; and the use of objects such as a balloon to graphically depict anger. In the balloon demonstration, first the balloon is blown up until, like anger, it bursts. Then another balloon is blown up taut but the air is slowly released. Demonstrating the value of each approach – where the outcome either leaves a shattered piece of rubber or a reusable balloon – provides a clear image which is readily transferable into a discussion of anger.

In addition to this dual approach the project also provides a follow-on weekly session just for the women who have completed the AWAKENS programme. Entitled 'Coping with kids', the focus of this group is to give the mother more control by helping her to regain confidence in her parenting skills.

Although to date the project has still to be formally evaluated, those concerned with it are convinced of its value in helping the child and mother to understand their experiences and in reducing acts of violence and aggression previously shown by the child.

KEY POINTS

☐   A lot more can be done to help service users to constructively express anger.

☐   As a nation we are not good at expressing anger constructively.

☐   Some techniques amount to no more than good old-fashioned common sense.

☐   Some techniques require knowledge and skilled workers.

☐   The positive expression of anger can identify triggers generating it.

☐   Expressing anger constructively can:

     – dissipate frustration,

     – identify the consequences of actions,

     – provide responsibility for actions,

     – help reduce aggression and violence.

REFERENCES

1 *Lost in Care* (2000) The Stationery Office (www.doh.gov.uk/lostincare/20102.htm).
2 *Learning the Lessons: The Report of the Tribunal of Inquiry into the Abuse of Children in Care in the Former County Council Areas of Gwynedd and Clwyd since 1974.* June 2000. The Stationery Office.
3 *No Secrets: Guidance on Developing Multi-Agency Policies and Procedures to Protect Vulnerable Adults from Abuse.* Available from website: www.doh.gov.uk\scg\nosecrets.htm
4 'On course for a change.' *Community Care.* 7 Aug. 1997.

KEY READING

George, M. 'Rooting it out.' *Community Care.* 14–20 Oct. 1999. One account of successful individual programme planning.
Dlyden, W. *Overcoming Anger.* Sheldon Press.
Ward, L. (ed.) (1999) *Innovations in Advocacy and Empowerment for People with Intellectual Disabilities.* Lisieux Ward.

Training material:
Williams, E. and Barlow, R. (2000) *Anger Control Training.* Winslow Press. A training pack providing a step-by-step guide to a cognitive/behavioural therapeutic approach to anger management.

BIBLIOGRAPHY

Books

Archer, J. and Browne, K. (1989) *Human Aggression*. Routledge.

Association of Directors of Social Services (1987) *Guidelines and Recommendations to Employers on Violence against Employees in the Personal Social Services*.

Balloch, S., McLean J. and Fisher, M. (eds) (1999) *Social Services: Working Under Pressure*. Policy Press.

Barker, M. (1981) *The New Racism: Conservatives and the Ideology of the Tribe*. Junction Books.

Barton, M. (2nd edn, 1997) *Ethnic and Racial Consciousness*. Longman.

Berkowitz, L. (1993) *Aggression*. University of Wisconsin, Madison.

Bishop, S. (1996) *Develop Your Assertiveness*. Kogan Page.

Booker, O. (1999) *Averting Aggression: Safety at Work with Adolescents and Adults*. Russell House Publishing.

Braham, P., Rattansi, A. and Skellington, R. (eds) (1992) *Racism and Anti-racism: Inequalities, Opportunities and Policies*. Sage.

Braithwaite, R. (1992) *Understanding Violence: Intervention and Prevention*. Radcliffe Professional Press.

British Association for People with Learning Disabilities (1996) *Physical Interventions: A Policy Framework*. BILD Publications.

The Children Act (1989) Guidance and Regulations (1991) Volume 4: Residential Care. HMSO.

Clifton, J. and Serdar, H. (2000) *Bully Off! Recognising and Tackling Workplace Bullying*. Russell House Publishing.

Coggans, N. (1995) *The Facts about Alcohol, Aggression and Adolescence*. Cassell.

Cohen, D. (1992) *Body Language in Relationships*. Sheldon Press.

Department of Health (1993) *Guidance on Permissible Forms of Control in Children's Residential Care*. HMSO. Information available at Department of Health website: www.doh.gov.uk

Department of Health (2000) *Draft Guidance on the Use of Physical Interventions for Staff Working with Children and Adults with Learning Disability and/or Autism*. www.doh.gov.uk/learningdisabilities/dgapp1.htm

Dlyden, W. *Overcoming Anger*. Sheldon Press.

East Sussex County Council. Social Services department. April 2000. *Restrictive Physical Interventions*.

Economic and Social Research Council (1998) *Taking Stock*. ESRC Violence Research Programme. Brunel University, Uxbridge, Middlesex UB8 3PH.

Field, T. (1996) *Bully in Sight*. Success Unlimited.

Green, R. G. (1990) *Human Aggression*. Open University Press.

Gullotta, T. P. and McElhaney, S. J. (eds) (1999) *Violence in Homes and Communities. Prevention, Intervention and Treatment*. National Mental Health Association. Sage.

Health and Safety Executive (1996) *Consulting Employees on Health and Safety: A Guide to the Law* INDG232 HSE Books (single copies free).

Health and Safety Executive (1998) *5 Steps to Risk Assessment* INDG163 (rev) HSE Books.

Health and Safety Executive (1998) *Working Alone in Safety* IND (G)73 (rev) HSE Books (single copies free).

Heller, R. (1998) *Managing Teams*. Dorling Kindersley.

Humphries, J. (1998) *Managing Successful Teams: How to Achieve Your Objectives by Working Effectively with Others*. How to Books.

Kirsta, A. (1994) *Deadlier than the Male: Violence and Aggression in Women*. Fontana.

Lawrence, C. (ed.) (1993) *The Security Journal*. Perpetuity Press.

Leadbetter, D. and Trewartha, R. (1999) *Handling Aggression and Violence at Work: A Training Manual*. Russell House Publishing.

Learning the Lessons: The Report of the Tribunal of Inquiry into the Abuse of Children in Care in the Former County Council Areas of Gwynedd and Clwyd since 1974. June 2000. The Stationery Office.

Lemon, C. (1997) *Assert Yourself*. Gower.

Lindenfield, G. (1993; rev. edn, 2000) *Managing Anger: Simple Steps to Dealing with Frustration and Threat*. Thorsons.

Lindenfield, G. (rev. edn, 2000) *Confident Children: Help Children Feel Good about Themselves*. Thorsons.

Lorenz, K. (1966) *On Aggression*. Methuen.

Lost in Care (2000) The Stationery Office. (www.doh.gov.uk/lostincare/20102.htm)

The Management of the Health and Safety Regulations (1999) The Stationery Office.

Morris, D. (1994) *Bodytalk: A World Guide to Gestures*. Cape.

No Secrets: Guidance on Developing Multi-Agency Policies and Procedures to Protect Vulnerable Adults from Abuse. Available from website: www.doh.gov.uk\scg\nosecrets.htm

Quilliam, S. (1994) *Child Watching: A Parents' Guide to Children's Body Language*. Ward Lock.

Sheldon, B. (1995) *Cognitive-behavioural Therapy: Research, Practice and Philosophy*. Routledge.

Smith, P. K. (1994) 'Social development', in A. M. Coleman (ed.) *Companion Encyclopaedia of Psychology*. Volume 2. Routledge, p. 731.

The Stephen Lawrence Inquiry. Report of an inquiry by Sir William Macpherson of Cluny. February 1999. The Stationery Office.

Storr, A. (1968) *Human Aggression*. Penguin.

Storr, A. (1991) *Human Destructiveness*. Routledge & Kegan Paul.

Taylor, G. (1999) *Managing Conflict*. Directory of Social Change, 24 Stevenson Way, London NW1 2DP.

Thompson, N. (1999) *Tackling Bullying and Harassment in the Workplace*. Pepar Publications.

Ward, L. (ed.) (1999) *Innovations in Advocacy and Empowerment for People with Intellectual Disabilities*. Lisieux Ward.

Webb, R. and Tossell, D. (1991) *Social Issues for Carers. A Community Care Perspective*. Edward Arnold.

Whittaker, D. Archer, L. and Hicks, L. (1998) *Working in Children's Homes: Challenges and Complexities*. Wiley.

Williams, E. and Barlow, R. (2000) *Anger Control Training*. Winslow Press.

Wilson, G. (1996) *Winning with Body Language*. Bloomsbury.

Articles

Braithwaite, R. 'Coming to terms with the effects of violence.' *Social Work Today*. 20 Oct. 1988.

Fletcher, K. 'Managing the media.' *Community Care*. 24 Feb.–1 March 2000.

George, M. 'Rooting it out.' *Community Care*. 14–20 Oct. 1999.

Hilton, A. and Roberts, J. 'Danger men at work.' *Community Care*. 22–28 April 1999.

Holihead, M. 'Whistleblowing.' *Community Care*. 20–26 Jan. 2000.

Huber, N. 'Black social workers still looking up at a glass ceiling.' *Community Care*. 14–20 Oct. 1999.

Hunter, M. 'How violence strikes.' *Community Care*. 29 July–4 Aug. 1999.

Hunter, M. 'Supporting front line staff.' *Community Care*. 5–11 Aug. 1999.

Hunter, M. 'Time to get a grip.' *Community Care*. 19–25 Aug. 1999.

No Fear Campaign: weekly contributed articles. *Community Care*. 22 July–Dec. 1999.

Pollard, J. 'Please sir, you're a bully.' *The Observer*. 2 April 2000.

Thompson, A. 'What happened to equality?' *Community Care*. 20–26 July 2000.

White, C. 'Keeping violence in mind.' *Community Care*. 28 Oct.–3 Nov. 1999.

'Workers in drugs case suffer zero tolerance.' News article. *Community Care*. 25 Nov.–1 Dec. 1999.

Information

Andrea Adams Trust is a UK national charity devoted to raising awareness of tackling bullying. Andrea Adams Trust, Maritime House, Basin Road North, Portslade, Brighton, East Sussex BN41 1WA (Tel: 01273 704900) email: aat@btinternet.com

BBC Education. Series of programmes shown on TV in 1998. BBC Education – *Bullying: A Survival Guide*. Information from: www.bbc.co.uk/education/archive/bully/

'Bullying at work' – survey report carried out on behalf of UNISON by Staffordshire University Business school in 1998. Published as a web page on: www.workdoctor.com/home/twd/employers/unison.html

Bully on line is an excellent website with lots of information provided by Tim Field and can be found at: www.successunlimited.co.uk/policy.htm

Criminal Injuries Compensation is available to individuals who have been subjected to assault. Information and forms for application can be obtained from: Criminal Injuries Compensation Authority, Tay House, 300 Bath Street, Glasgow G2 4lN (Tel: 0141 331 2726).

Useful websites for information about ethnic issues:
www.blink.org.uk
www.kingsfund.org.uk

The Commission for Racial Equality operates from: 10–12 Allington Street, London SW1E 5EH (Tel: 0207 828 7022). They will also have the number of your local Racial Equality Council.

University of Exeter: 'Policy on the protection of dignity at work and study'. This policy statement is available to be viewed at: www.ex.ac.uk/EAD/personnel/ppdws.htm

GPMU Campaign: 'Bullying – spotting the signs'. Website: www.gpmu.org.uk/bullysign.html

National Institute for Social Work Briefing Number 26: 'Violence against social care workers'. This briefing gives an overview of the literature on violence and abuse of staff, the findings from NISW Workforce Studies on violence, and local authority and other organisational policies and guidelines. Price £1.75, October 1999, from NISW, 5 Tavistock Place, London WC1H 9SN. Website: www.nisw.org.uk or info@nisw.org.uk 3

A Safer Place: Combating Violence Against Social Care Staff. Report of the Task Force and National Action Plan. Department of Health. The National Task Force on Violence Against

Social Care Staff was established following the death of Jenny Morrison who was killed by a service user in November 1998. The website contains comprehensive information for employees and employers: www.doh.gov.uk/violencetaskforce

UNISON campaign: 'Bullying at work'. Details from: www.unison.org.uk/
The independent consumer guide *Which?* magazine carried out a product test on personal alarms in December 1994. Further information may be obtained from: Which? Ltd, Consumers Association, 2 Marylebone Road, London NW1 4DF (website: www.which.net).

The Institute of Conflict Management is a not for profit organisation whose remit is to investigate ways of developing nationally recognised standards in the fields of conflict management and prevention in the workplace. Information may be obtained from: The Institute of Conflict Management, 840 Melton Road, Thurmaston, Leicester, Leicestershire. LE4 8BN (website: www.conflictmanagement.org).

The Suzy Lamplugh Trust is a registered charity whose aim is to create a safer society. The Trust provides training, information and publications in personal safety. Information from: The Suzy Lamplugh Trust, 14 East Sheen Avenue, London SW14 8AS.

INDEX